WU120 AST

KU-242-445

16786 21 DEC 89

Disease, Drugs and the Dentist

Second edition

Disease, Drugs and the Dentist

Second edition

Humphrey D. Astley Hope, MB, BS, BDS, DOrth
General Dental Practitioner and previously Dental Surgeon to Newbury District Hospital

and

Michael D. Hellier, MA, MB, BCh, FRCP, MD
Consultant Physician, Princess Margaret Hospital, Swindon

WRIGHT
London Boston Singapore Sydney Toronto Wellington

Wright
is an imprint of Butterworth Scientific

 PART OF REED INTERNATIONAL P.L.C.

All rights reserved. No part of this publication may be reproduced or transmitted in any form or by any means, including photocopying and recording, without the written permission of the copyright holder, application for which should be addressed to the Publishers, or in accordance with the provisions of the Copyright Act 1956 (as amended), or under the terms of any licence permitting limited copying issued by the Copyright Licensing Agency, 7 Ridgmount Street, London WC1E 7AE, England. Such written permission must also be obtained before any part of this publication is stored in a retrieval system of any nature.

Any person who does any unauthorized act in relation to this publication may be liable to criminal prosecution and civil claims for damages.

This book is sold subject to the Standard Conditions of Sale of Net Books and may not be re-sold in the UK below the net price given by the Publishers in their current price list.

First published by John Wiley and Sons, 1982
Second edition 1989

© **Butterworth & Co. (Publishers) Ltd, 1989**

British Library Cataloguing in Publication Data
Astley Hope, Humphrey D.
Disease, drugs and the dentist.—2nd ed.
1. Drugs. Action – For dentistry
I. Title II. Hellier, Michael D.
615′.7′0246176
ISBN 0–7236–0955–1

Library of Congress Cataloging in Publication Data
Hope, Humphrey D. Astley (Humphrey Dugdale Astley)
Disease, drugs, and the dentist / by Humphrey D. Astley Hope and Michael D. Hellier. – 2nd ed.
p. cm.
ISBN 0–7236–0955–1 :
1. Diseases. 2. Drugs. 3. Dentists. 4. Oral manifestations of general diseases. 5. Drugs–Side effects. I. Hellier, Michael D. II. Title.
[DNLM: 1. Dentistry. 2. Disease. 3. Drugs. QV 50 H791d]
RC48.H64 1989
616—dc 19
DNLM/DLC
for Library of Congress 88–8133
CIP

L. H. M. C.
LIBRARY
ACCESSION No.
50986

Typeset by Latimer Trend & Company Ltd, Plymouth
Printed and bound by Hartnolls Ltd, Bodmin, Cornwall

Preface to second edition

Since this book appeared in print 5 years ago, several new disease entities have been recognized, new drugs developed and new treatment regimens put into practice. Where these have a bearing on dentistry, they have been incorporated into this new edition and at the same time the authors have enlarged the text in response to criticisms or suggestions relating to the original.

With grateful thanks we acknowledge assistance from Dr Brian Greenwood CBE of the Medical Research Council and Dr Dionne Smythe of Paddington Green Children's Hospital. Professor W.H. Binnie of Baylor College of Dentistry, Dallas has again given help with drugs commonly used in the USA.

Without the diligence of Mrs Linda Totten, the typescript would never have reached the publishers and once again we acknowledge the assistance and forbearance of our patient wives.

Preface to first edition

This little book is written as an 'aide memoire', primarily for the general dental practitioner. In no way should it be considered as a texbook of oral medicine or even a manual of oral signs of general disease. It is designed to assist the dentist when confronted with a patient who tells him/her that he suffers from a certain condition and is under treatment with such and such a drug.

The contents have been laid out alphabetically in three sections. The first lists diseases and conditions likely to be encountered, and the third drugs which the patient may be taking. The former are given under their proper (medical) titles, with their colloquial names cross-referenced to them. The drugs in the latter section are set out under their pharmacological titles with proprietary names (GB and US) similarly cross-referenced. For the sake of brevity the lists are far from complete. Primary diseases of the teeth and gums have been omitted, as it was felt that the readers would be as conversant with these as the authors. The selection is based on three principles: firstly, diseases of which the sufferers may be at hazard in the course of dental treatment either by reason of the disease itself or its treatment; secondly, communicable diseases where special precautions should be taken to protect dentist, staff and other patients; and lastly, a general group with or without oral manifestations, whose names may crop up in taking a medical history.

As in other books of this type, a number of statements are based on the opinion of the authors and are not substantiated by proof. As an example, we advise the use of a local anaesthetic without adrenaline in patients with certain cardiovascular conditions. Research has not demonstrated any dangerous rise in blood adrenaline following the extravascular injection of a local anaesthetic with adrenaline in reasonable quantity. However, aspirating syringes are only as foolproof as the hand that holds them, and, while the effects of intravenous prilocaine and felypressin on a damaged human heart have not been investigated, we feel that this alternative or lignocaine alone would be less dangerous than a local anaesthetic containing adrenaline under these circumstances.

The authors have done their best to supply United States equivalents of drugs used in Great Britain, but in a few instances no equivalent is listed, and, no doubt, there are other situations where a drug is used in the United States and not here. In such a wide and complex field, there will be omissions and errors resulting from recent study with which we are unacquainted, but we hope these are not of sufficient magnitude to seriously mislead a dentist consulting the book for guidance.

An index and list of references have been omitted to conserve space, but readers are advised to refer to standard textbooks of General and Dental Medicine in situations where they wish to find out more about the subject.

The authors wish to thank professional colleagues whom they have consulted during the preparation of this book, particularly Professor W.H. Binnie of Baylor College of Dentistry, Dallas; Mr John Fieldhouse of the Department of Oral Surgery, Princess Margaret Hospital, Swindon and Dr Patrick Smythe of St John's Road, Newbury. We acknowledge with gratitude advice and assistance from Dr John Jarvis of John Wiley & Sons on the presentation of the script. Both of us owe a great debt to our secretaries, Mrs Jacqueline Birch, Miss Sharon Brain, and Mrs Doreen Burnup who have coped uncomplaining with sheaves of barely legible handwriting, and to our two patient wives who have supplied both material help and encouragement.

In conclusion we should like to thank Professor Brian Cooke, Dean of the Dental School, University of Wales whose suggestion initiated this book and who checked through our manuscripts at the end. It might be said that he abetted procreation and was midwife to delivery.

Contents

Preface to second edition v
Preface to first edition vi

Section 1

Alphabetical list of diseases and conditions 1

Section 2

Weights, measures and normal values 211

Section 3

Alphabetical list of pharmacological and proprietary drug names 215

Section 1
Alphabetical list of diseases and conditions

A

A

ACHALASIA

This is a disturbance of the swallowing mechanism due to denervation of the lower oesophagus, which is unable to relax during swallowing. The oesophageal musculature above this level hypertrophies and the oesophagus progressively dilates. The aetiology is unknown. As the condition progresses food accumulates in the oesophagus and putrefies. The mucosa becomes inflamed and, in approximately 5% of people, carcinoma of the oesophagus occurs. A more common complication is lung aspiration with progressive pulmonary disease. The condition occurs in either sex, at any age. Pain is a frequent presenting feature, sometimes mimicking angina and occurs in 80% of people. Dysphagia and regurgitation, often of foul-smelling food remnants, become progressively more severe and are accompanied by weight loss.

The diagnosis is made by barium swallow. Drug treatment has little to offer, although occasional inhalation of *octyl nitrate* can relieve the pain of oesophageal spasm.

The treatment of choice is surgery. The circular muscle layer of the lower oesophagus is cut (Heller's operation). Alternative treatment is rupture of the circular muscle layer by balloon dilatation.

Dental significance

Because regurgitation of solid matter can occur many hours after the last meal, general anaesthesia is a hazard. If essential for dental treatment, it should be carried out by intubation with a cuffed tube. The possibility of underlying lung disease must be borne in mind. Achalasia should be remembered as a cause of halitosis when no oral or pulmonary disease is present to account for it.

ACHONDROPLASIA

This hereditary failure in the ossification of bones formed in cartilage, appears in fetal life. Those who survive are the circus dwarfs with short limbs and large heads. There is no treatment, but apart from the bone deformity health and life expectation are normal.

Dental significance

Growth of the mandible is unaffected but that of the middle third of the face is deficient. This results in a class III malocclusion, but the teeth themselves are usually normal. Intubation can be difficult if required for general anaesthesia.

ACNE VULGARIS

This condition usually commences at puberty and is due to overactivity of the sebaceous glands. The main distribution is on the face, central chest and back, the areas of highest sebum production. The sex incidence is equal. Hyperkeratosis and inspissation of sebum in the follicles cause the primary lesion of acne, the comedo or blackhead. An inflammatory response may produce sterile pus forming a pustule.

Mild peeling agents such as sulphur and salicylic acid are useful treatment. *Benzoyl peroxide* as a cream or lotion may be beneficial. Long-term use of antibiotics by mouth may be very effective, *tetracycline* being the antibiotic of choice. Exposure on a regular basis to ultraviolet light, either natural or by lamp, is advocated.

Dental significance

There is no dental significance. Because the condition is one of adolescence, most of the dentition is spared pigmentation from long-term *tetracycline* treatment. Cervical margins of second molars and wisdom teeth are all that are likely to be affected.

ACRODERMATITIS ENTEROPATHICA

This is a persistent dermatitis affecting the perioral area and peripheries, commencing with vesicles which progress to crusting, thickening and, sometimes, secondary infection. Two-thirds of patients have a family history. Plasma zinc levels are low and the condition responds dramatically to treatment with zinc supplements. It may be confused with psoriasis or candidiasis.

Dental significance

Abnormalities of taste, oedema, desquamation and ulceration of the oral mucosa may be seen in addition to weeping erosions at the corners of the mouth. The condition is not infectious.

ACROMEGALY

Excess of growth hormone, which in young life results in gigantism, causes acromegaly after the epiphyses have closed. It is produced by an acidophil tumour of the anterior pituitary gland. A large jaw, coarse skin and spade-like hands are the special features. Muscle weakness, defective vision and diabetes are not uncommon.

Treatment is by surgical removal of the tumour or irradiation. *Bromocriptine* is used to suppress high levels of growth hormone.

Dental significance

The skeletal discrepancies between maxilla and mandible are gross and any correction, after eradication of the tumour, will require surgery.

General anaesthetics should only be administered in hospital and even then, not entertained lightly. Apart from the incidence of diabetes mellitus and other defects, the physical deformity of the mouth can make intubation very difficult.

ACTINOMYCOSIS

This rare bacterial infection, which occurs chiefly in males between 20 and 30, affects the body in one of three sites: the cervicofacial area, the ileocaecal part of the intestines or the lungs. In each it produces a hard mass of tissue which eventually breaks down and discharges through multiple sinuses.

It is treated by high doses of *penicillin* over a long period and by surgery.

Dental significance

The cervicofacial area is the commonest site, where the condition usually presents as a hard nodular swelling at the angle of the jaw. The skin which is bound to it is blue–red and multiple sinuses develop discharging pus which may show to the naked eye the characteristic yellow granules. There is often trismus. Bone involvement is rare unless there has been a recent fracture or extraction, and the lymph glands are seldom swollen without secondary infection.

Microscopical examination of the pus will usually show the pseudomycelia of the bacteria and clinch the diagnosis.

ADDISON'S DISEASE

For Addison's disease, *see under* Adrenal diseases.

ADRENAL DISEASES

The adrenal gland is composed of an outer cortex and central medulla. The cortex secretes the following hormones: mineralocorticoids, mainly aldosterone; glucocorticoids, cortisol and corticosterone; androgens and, to a lesser extent, progesterone and oestrone.

The medulla produces two hormones: adrenaline and noradrenaline.

The following conditions result from over-activity of the adrenal gland: Cushing's syndrome, primary hyperaldosteronism (Conn's syndrome) and phaeochromocytoma. The condition resulting from under-activity is Addison's disease.

Cushing's syndrome

This condition results from over-activity of the adrenal cortex and may be due to hyperplasia or to benign or malignant tumours. The features of the condition are due to excessive glucocorticoid production, causing obesity with a characteristic distribution of fat over the neck and trunk but sparing the arms and legs. The face becomes rounded with a high colour. Acne, hirsutism and amenorrhoea occur in women, and impotence in men. Other symptoms include weakness, bruising, backache and symptoms of the complications of Cushing's syndrome – hypertension, diabetes and depression. The treatment of an adenoma or carcinoma is surgical. Treatment of bilateral adrenal hyperplasia is controversial and may be surgical: adrenalectomy with or without pituitary irradiation and hormone replacement. Medical adrenalectomy may be produced with certain enzyme-blocking drugs.

Patients who have been treated by adrenalectomy will be on a maintenance dose of cortisone. This will require supplementing for surgery (*see* Addison's disease).

Primary hyperaldosteronism (Conn's syndrome)

This condition results from a defect in the adrenal cortex leading to increased aldosterone production and resulting in hypertension and hypokalaemia. The latter may produce muscle weakness, paraesthesia, tetany, polyuria and thirst.

Treatment may be surgical with adrenalectomy or medical using aldosterone antagonists.

Phaeochromocytoma

This is a tumour of the adrenal medulla producing excessive quantities of adrenaline and noradrenaline. This causes paroxysmal or persistent hypertension. In the paroxysmal type, the patient may describe episodes when he or she experiences a feeling of apprehension, palpitations, excessive sweating, flushing, epigastric fullness and headaches. Treatment where possible is surgical with removal of the tumour. If this is not possible, for example an inoperable malignant tumour, hypertension is controlled with α- or β-adrenergic blocking drugs.

Dental significance

Dental treatment of patients with over-activity of the adrenal glands must be approached with caution. Hypertension and blood vessel fragility increases the danger of bruising and haemorrhage following surgery. Osteoporosis weakens the bones and fracture of the maxillary tuberosity or the mandible can occur at the time of extractions. Diabetes is an added complication (*see* Diabetes mellitus). General anaesthetics are to be avoided or given in hospital.

Addison's disease

This condition most commonly results from autoimmune adrenalitis or tuberculosis. The clinical features result from loss of cortisol and aldosterone. The condition is more common in women than men and may have been present for years before the diagnosis is made. The prevalence is approximately 1 in 25 000 of the population. The main signs and symptoms are tiredness, weakness, anorexia and nausea. Pigmentation due to excess adrenocorticotrophin (ACTH) and melanocyte stimulating hormone (MSH) production is characteristic, being prominent inside the cheeks, on the gums and lips. Vomiting, weight loss, dizziness and postural hypotension are other common features.

Of great importance is the fact that patients with Addison's disease may be asymptomatic until stressed by intercurrent illness when they may become acutely ill with vomiting and severe hypotension (addisonian crisis).

Treatment is with *cortisone*, usually 20 mg in the morning and 10 mg at night.

Major surgery requires parenteral treatment, *hydrocortisone succinate* 100 mg i.m. every 6 hours, starting with the premedication and continuing for 72 hours or until the patient is able to take cortisone by mouth. The above procedure also applies to minor surgery but followed for 24 hours only. Very minor procedures may be covered by *hydrocortisone succinate* 100 mg i.m.

Treatment of adrenal crisis

In this serious event *hydrocortisone* 100 mg i.m. should be given immediately and an intravenous infusion established, with further *hydrocortisone* 100 mg i.v. One litre of physiological saline plus *glucose* 50 g is given intravenously over half an hour, followed by 2–4 litres over 24 hours. *Hydrocortisone* 100 mg i.v. is given every 4 hours.

Dental significance

Brown patches of recent onset on the buccal mucosa and gingiva in non-pigmented races may be the first indication of Addison's disease, and should be reported.

At least 200 mg of *hydrocortisone* for injection should be carried in every dental surgery. It should be checked frequently to make sure it is not out of date, and dental assistants should be taught how to mix and prepare it for injection.

Patients with adrenocortical insufficiency, being treated with *cortisone*, will require additional *cortisone* when surgery or general anaesthetics are contemplated. If no more than a simple extraction under local anaesthesia, it is sufficient for the patient to double the morning dose of *cortisone*, *hydrocortisone* by injection being readily available (100 mg i.v.) should there be any evidence of hypotensive collapse. General anaesthetics and more extensive surgery are best carried out in hospital under controlled replacement therapy as described.

Adrenal insufficiency

If within the previous 12 months any patients have been treated with *cortisone* in excess of 5 mg daily for more than a week, subsequent adrenocortical insufficiency must be suspected. With approval of their doctor they should be given *prednisolone* 5 mg three times daily for 2 days starting the day prior to surgery and then the dosage reduced by 5 mg a day over the following 3 days. Soluble *hydrocortisone* must be available.

AGAMMAGLOBULINAEMIA

A wide variety of immunodeficiency disorders is now recognized. X-linked infantile agammaglobulinaemia (Bruton type) is a disease in which B-lymphocytes and plasma cells are absent, resulting in gross deficiency of immunoglobulins. Cell-mediated immunity is normal. This deficiency results in recurrent infections to which there is minimal resistance with consequent rapid spread of infection if untreated. Response to appropriate antibiotics is usually good. Treatment of Bruton type and other immunodeficiencies involves early detection and intensive treatment of infective episodes and injections of γ-globulin at frequent intervals.

Dental significance

Strict attention to oral hygiene is of utmost importance. Extractions must be carried out under antibiotic cover.

AGRANULOCYTOSIS AND NEUTROPENIA

Neutropenia is a reduction of white blood cells below the level of $2500/mm^3$. Agranulocytosis is complete or almost complete absence of neutrophils. The causes are multiple and include drugs, leukaemias, aplastic anaemia and hyposplenism.

In practice symptoms are uncommon with a count of $1000–1500/mm^3$ and common below $500/mm^3$.

Acute neutropenia

Symptoms vary in their severity depending on the acuteness of onset. They may be divided into:

1. Constitutional symptoms, chills, sweats, headaches, muscle pains and exhaustion.
2. Infective symptoms due to invasion of the mucous membranes and skin by bacteria. Lesions in the mouth are most prominent, sore throats, reddening of the throat, progressing to ulceration and mucosal necrosis. Ulcers occur on the gums, lips, buccal mucous membranes, throat and pharynx. The ulcers are often extremely painful. Necrotic ulceration of the skin also occurs.

Chronic neutropenia

1. Constitutional symptoms are less severe (infections frequently involve the skin). Fatigue, lassitude and weakness may be independent of any infection or anaemia.
2. Infectious symptoms. Recurrent infections are the dominant feature of chronic neutropenia, being prolonged, slow healing and resistant to treatment. Infections of the mouth and throat are more common.

Treatment involves prevention and management of established neutropenia where possible, e.g. withdrawal of causative drug and treatment of complications with appropriate antibiotic therapy.

In the chronic form treatment mainly involves prevention and treatment of infection.

Dental significance

Recurrent ulcerative and haemorrhagic gingivitis, often associated with destructive periodontal disease, may be the first sign of this condition, and a patient seen with these manifestations should be referred for a white blood cell count without delay. Surgery should be put off if possible, but if extractions are unavoidable they must be carried out under strict antibiotic cover.

AIDS (ACQUIRED IMMUNE DEFICIENCY SYNDROME)

This is a contagious disease caused by a retrovirus, the human immunodeficiency virus (HIV, but previously designated HTLV-III or LAV). It has a long, silent incubation period, usually lasting several years, resulting in a slowly progressive disease which is inevitably lethal. Within 5 years of infection, 25% of people develop AIDS and it now seems probable that all people infected with the virus will ultimately die of the disease. Unlike most viral infections, antibodies to the virus fail to neutralize or eliminate the virus and thus provide no immunity.

The diagnosis of AIDS is made when a disease indicative of underlying cellular immune deficiency (such as Kaposi's sarcoma or a severe opportunistic infection) occurs in someone with no known cause of reduced resistance reported to be associated with that disease. The following opportunistic infections are considered moderately predictive of underlying cellular immune deficiency: intestinal cryptosporidiosis, pneumocystis, toxoplasmosis, aspergillosis or cryptococcosis. Also suspect are oesophagitis due to candidiasis, viral infections such as cytomegalovirus, herpes simplex when causing widespread involvement and progressive multifocal leukoencephalopathy presumed to be caused by papovavirus.

The main at-risk group is that of the male homosexual/bisexual population who make up approximately 90% of the established cases of AIDS. Also at risk are drug takers sharing syringes and needles, the heterosexual contacts of infected individuals and infants of infected mothers. A number of haemophiliac patients contracted the infection when receiving imported factor VIII. At the time of writing, spread through normal heterosexual intercourse appears to be rare in the UK.

AIDS is a blood-borne infection spread by inoculation of infected blood or blood products. There is no evidence that the virus is spread by oral or respiratory routes, casual personal contact or airborne droplets. The following modes of transmission are particularly relevant to medical and nursing staff:

1. Direct percutaneous inoculation of infected blood.

2. Spillage of infected blood to abraded or damaged epithelial surfaces.
3. Contamination of mucosal surfaces (i.e. accidental splash in eyes).

AIDS-related complex (ARC) is a persistent generalized lymphadenopathy (PGL) or pre-AIDS syndrome. It is defined as lymphadenopathy at two or more non-inguinal sites for 3 months or longer plus one of the following: weight loss, fever, diarrhoea, fatigue or night sweats, and certain markers of immune deficiency.

Kaposi's sarcoma – in Europe, this is due to an indolent vascular spindle cell proliferation involving the skin, especially in the peripheries. Initially, it may appear as a localized red or purple, flat or raised lesion looking like a bruise or angioma. Nodal and visceral involvement may supervene. It is frequently found as part of the AIDS syndrome.

At present there is no specific treatment for AIDS and no curative drug is likely in the foreseeable future because, once infected, the viral genetic code is inserted into the human cellular genetic code. However, recent studies in the USA using the antiviral agent *zidovudine* (AZT, Retrovir$_{GB}$) have demonstrated an improvement in survival of AIDS sufferers and the drug is now approved in the USA and the UK.

Dental significance

Infection with HIV can be transmitted in the dental surgery to either the dentist and his assistant or to another patient. While at the time of writing there is no vaccine to offer protection, it is at least cheering to appreciate that the virus is far less robust than that of hepatitis B and the infectivity considerably less. In addition to being present in the blood, the virus can be found in the saliva of an infected person, as well as other body fluids, but it would seem that the transmission of a significant amount of infected blood into the dentist, his staff or another patient is the only likely means of spread in the dental surgery. A follow-up of many cases of needlestick injuries in dentists has only shown one recipient to become seropositive.

High-risk patients are homosexuals, drug addicts, haemophiliacs and their sexual partners, together with children born to infected mothers. However, the dentist can never be sure whether the patient he is treating is clear of infection and strict precautions should be taken. All instruments which are put in the mouth should be either disposable or should be sterilized in an autoclave at a minimum of 134°C for 3 minutes, working surfaces which might be contaminated with blood or saliva should be disinfected with hypochlorite solution or 2% glutaraldehyde, and the dentist and his assistant should wear a face mask, eye protection and preferably operating gloves. A safe procedure for replacing needles in their sheaths and disposing of sharps is essential. It is not in the domain of the dentist to take blood for, or arrange a test for, HIV antibody as the implications of being seropositive are so sinister for the patient. If there are serious grounds for suspecting the condition, the patient should be advised to consult his doctor for an examination and the dentist should let the doctor know of his suspicions in confidence.

Oral manifestations are among the earliest signs of AIDS. They consist of oral candidiasis, which is present in 70% of sufferers, hairy leukoplakia on the sides of the tongue and herpes simplex, which is often more severe, more persistent and erupting in unusual sites. As the disease progresses the purplish elevated patches of Kaposi's sarcoma may be found in the mouth, notably on the palate and immune deficiency periodontitis can develop.

Candidiasis should be treated with *nystatin* (Nystan pastilles) four times daily or *miconazole* (Daktarin oral gel_{GB}) 5 ml held in the mouth and then swallowed four times daily or, if very severe, *ketoconazole* ($Nizoral_{GB,US}$) 400 mg daily, but this should only be used in conjunction with the patient's doctor as it is necessary to monitor liver function when prescribing it. There is no treatment for hairy leukoplakia, but the eruptions of herpes simplex can be helped by the topical application of *acyclovir* (Zovirax $cream_{GB,US}$) five times daily or *acyclovir* by mouth (Zovirax $Tabs_{GB,US}$) 200 mg five times daily. For the periodontitis which is accompanied by considerable bone loss and mobility of teeth, hand scaling should be instituted together with irrigation or mouthwashes of 0.2% *chlorhexidine* ($Corsodyl_{GB}$, $Peridex_{US}$). Peroxide should be avoided.

Persistent aphthous ulcers may also be a problem and cause great discomfort, requiring a *benzocaine* lozenge ($Merocaine_{GB}$) before meals, and xerostomia, usually secondary to treatment, may require the prescription of an artificial saliva ($Glandosane_{GB}$) to be used as required.

As infection with cytomegalovirus is a common association, pregnant female staff should not assist at treatment.

ALBERS-SCHÖNBERG DISEASE

For Albers-Schönberg disease, *see* Osteopetrosis.

ALCOHOLISM

An alcoholic may be considered as an individual who habitually drinks an excessive amount of alcohol or who has special problems relating to consumption of alcohol. Not all alcoholics develop the medical complications of alcohol and, conversely, alcohol-induced disease may occur in non-alcoholics.

Addiction is the stage of physical dependence on alcohol and leads to disintegration of social status and personality. Symptoms include memory blanks following drinking sessions, restlessness if without alcohol, tremor, morning retching, vomiting and night sweating. Cessation of alcohol results in withdrawal syndromes. The early stage (6–8 hours) includes tremulousness, nausea, retching and sweating. The late stage (after 48 hours) is the syndrome of delirium tremens, i.e. mental confusion, disorientation, restlessness, fear, paranoia, hallucinations and, occasionally, epilepsy.

Opinions vary as to the dangerous level of daily alcohol intake but most authorities agree that a sustained level of 3–4 units a day in men and 2–3 units in women (where a unit is equivalent to half a pint of beer or a glass of wine) is liable to lead to serious physical harm. However, considerable individual variation in susceptibility to alcohol damage exists.

The physical consequences of alcohol are legion. Accidents commonly result from intoxication and head trauma is frequent. Acute pancreatitis with a high mortality rate complicates high alcohol intake, also gastritis and gastric erosions which may result in haematemesis. There is an increased risk of vascular disease, cardiomyopathy and tendency to a rise in blood pressure. Liver damage is the most well-known complication of alcohol abuse. Initially, changes are reversible but once cirrhosis is established the damage persists and progresses accompanied by the fearsome complications of portal hypertension, variceal haemorrhage and carcinoma of the liver. Apart from the psychoses associated with alcohol withdrawal, alcohol causes cerebral atrophy, dementia, Korsakoff's psychosis and Wernicke's encephalopathy. Malnutrition in association with high alcohol consumption may result in wet and dry beri-beri. Peripheral neuropathy occurs in 10% and suicides are much commoner among alcoholics.

Prevention is of the utmost importance for once alcoholism is established very few alcoholics are ever cured. At-risk groups need identifying and advising. Management of the addict includes management of the physical problems and withdrawal syndromes together with techniques to promote abstinence. 'Drying out' is often best carried out in hospital. Promotion of abstinence necessitates a change in attitude best brought about by the help of self-help groups such as 'AA' (Alcoholics Anonymous) and hospital self-help groups. At-risk occupations such as bar-person or publican should be changed. Living in a therapeutic community such as a hostel for alcoholics may help. Drugs such as *disulfiram* (Antabuse$_{GB, US}$) have only a limited part to play.

Dental significance

Most dentists will be more than familiar with the smell of alcohol on the breath and know that even in mid-morning this is not diagnostic of an alcoholic. Oral manifestations of alcoholism result from associated vitamin deficiency, and are likely to include glossitis, angular cheilitis and, sometimes, candida infection and leukoplakia. *Aspirin* is liable to cause gastric irritation, and *paracetamol* should be prescribed as an alternative analgesic, but avoiding large doses. Because of the possibility of incipient liver damage, narcotic analgesics and hypnotics should be avoided and *diazepam* (Valium$_{GB, US}$) used in reduced dosage. *Penicillin* is the safest antibiotic. General anaesthetics are a hazard, and *lignocaine* should be used with restraint. *Metronidazole* (Flagyl$_{GB, US}$) must not be prescribed for patients who are alcoholics and especially for those who are being treated with *disulfiram* (Antabuse$_{GB, US}$).

Oral carcinoma is said to be more common in alcoholics, and the floor of the mouth should be carefully examined for this.

ALKAPTONURIA

This is a rare hereditary disorder resulting from the absence of the enzyme homogentisic acid oxidase. Because of this defect, homogentisic acid accumulates in cartilage, connective tissue and urine, giving rise to a degenerative arthritis of the spine and larger peripheral joints.

Dental significance

Pigmentation of the teeth has been reported.

ALLERGIC RHINITIS

This condition, popularly called hay fever, results from allergy to one of the grass pollens or to a multitude of other allergens such as household dust, feathers or fur. Desensitizing injections prior to its occurrence are often successful when the condition is seasonal or the allergen can be identified. In an attack antihistamines, such as *chlorpheniramine* (Piriton$_{GB}$) 4 mg twice daily, are helpful, but suit some individuals better than others. Nebulizers containing *sodium cromoglycate* (Rynacrom$_{GB}$) or *beclomethasone* (Beconase$_{GB}$) are also of value.

Dental significance

When possible dentistry should be avoided during attacks. The nasal obstruction is a complicating factor to general anaesthetics and, for sufferers, these are best planned for when the condition is not prevalent. If a general anaesthetic is necessary at short notice, the patient's doctor should be consulted with regards to a short course of *cortisone* (*cortisone acetate* 10 mg three times daily) to suppress the symptoms.

ALZHEIMER'S DISEASE

The cause of this rapidly progressive dementia is obscure, but it may result from a defect in the earliest stage of protein synthesis. Widespread neuronal degeneration produces an appearance of the cell known as neurofibrillary tangle. Earliest signs are loss of short-term memory followed by inability to reason, impairment of speech, intellectual failure, inability to read, increasing helplessness and death in about 5 years. There is no specific treatment, but improvement has been reported with use of the cholinergic drug *tetrahydro-amino acridine* (THA).

Dental significance

In many ways, this miserable disease is quite as distressing for relatives as it is for its victims. The dentist should be aware of its name and nature to save the embarrassment of explanations. Treatment must be adjusted to that with which the patient can cooperate, bearing in mind the prognosis.

AMYLOIDOSIS

This is the name given to a group of conditions where protein/polysaccharide complexes are laid down in tissue. These may be divided into two main groups:

1. Primary amyloid, associated with plasma cell dyscrasia and overt myeloma, affecting predominantly the tongue, heart, gastrointestinal tract, muscle, ligaments and skin.
2. Secondary amyloid, associated with chronic infections and rheumatoid arthritis, affecting liver, spleen, kidney and adrenal.

A mixed pattern of (1) and (2) may occur in approximately 30% of cases.

Clinical manifestations of primary amyloid are cardiac, gastrointestinal with malabsorption, bleeding and diarrhoea, neuropathies, skin involvement with subcutaneous haemorrhage and purpura, macroglossia, xerostomia and dysphagia.

Clinical manifestations of secondary amyloid are hepatosplenomegaly, renal and hepatic impairment, oedema and nephrotic syndrome.

Dental significance

The enlarged tongue is firm and shows indentations on the edges where it rests against the teeth. Mobility is reduced, which may result in speech impairment and poor oral hygiene. Patients should be instructed to clean their teeth efficiently after each meal as the tongue is unable to assist in this function.

Orthostatic hypotension is a common symptom and dentists who work on supine patients should elevate them from the horizontal slowly.

ANAEMIA

This is defined as a reduction in the concentration of haemoglobin in the peripheral blood below the normal, 13.5 g/100 ml in men, 11.5 g/100 ml in women. Anaemia may result from: blood loss, impaired red blood cell formation, and increased red blood cell destruction. The main types in these groups will be described.

Iron deficiency anaemia

This is the commonest type of anaemia. It occurs in all ages but most commonly in women of childbearing age. The major causes are excessive menstrual blood loss, gastrointestinal haemorrhage and, occasionally, deficient diet or impaired iron absorption.

Besides general tiredness, nails may become brittle and spoon shaped, papillae on the tongue atrophy, resulting in a smooth pale tongue, which may become red and sore. Rarely leukoplakia of the tongue occurs. Angular stomatitis with soreness and cracking at the angle of the mouth is common. A syndrome of iron deficiency anaemia, dysphagia and glossitis (the Plummer–Vinson syndrome) is seen in middle-aged women, the dysphagia resulting from a fine web in the postcricoid region of the oesophagus. It is important to establish the cause of the anaemia and to exclude serious underlying gastrointestinal disease. Treatment involves management of the underlying cause and iron supplements, usually oral, occasionally parenteral. Transfusion may be necessary where the anaemia is severe.

Dental significance

Iron deficiency anaemia is common and is probably present in a tenth of the female population. The oral manifestations (atrophic glossitis, angular stomatitis, candidiasis and sometimes aphthous ulceration) may be the presenting symptoms. When seen, the dentist should be alert to the likely underlying pathology, which can be confirmed by a blood picture.

Treatment is by oral *ferrous sulphate* or *ferrous fumarate* (Fersa-mal$_{GB}$, Ferancee$_{US}$) 200 mg three times daily after meals, and the patient's doctor should be informed so he can check there is no hidden cause of the anaemia. There are no contraindications to routine dentistry, but treatment of the anaemia should be instituted before planning multiple extractions or oral surgery.

The oxygen-carrying capacity of the blood is reduced by the condition, and general anaesthesia should be conducted with a high concentration of oxygen in the anaesthetic gases to guard against cerebral anoxia. With haemoglobin levels below 10 g/100 ml, general anaesthesia should be postponed.

Megaloblastic anaemias

These constitute 5% of all anaemias and are caused by lack of vitamin B_{12}, folate or both. The name derives from the appearance of the bone marrow.

Vitamin B_{12} deficiency gives rise to the following clinical manifestations: megaloblastic anaemia, glossitis, and peripheral neuritis and subacute combined degeneration of the spinal cord.

The causes are:

1. Dietary deficiency, rare in this country except in strict vegetarians.
2. Intestinal disorders:
   (*a*) addisonian pernicious anaemia results from a failure of the gastric antrum to produce intrinsic factor, which is essential for ileal absorption of vitamin B_{12};
   (*b*) bacterial contamination of the gut interfering with vitamin B_{12} absorption;
   (*c*) ileal disease (e.g. Crohn's);
   (*d*) surgical resection of the ileum.

A blood picture will reveal fewer red blood cells which are larger and contain full amounts of haemoglobin giving rise to the typical macrocytic normochromic anaemia with an increased mean corpuscular volume (MCV) and normal mean corpuscular haemoglobin concentration (MCHC). The white blood count and platelet count are frequently low and the polymorphonuclear cells show hypersegmentation of the nucleus.

It is of the utmost importance to establish the diagnosis before neurological complications occur as these may be irreversible.

Treatment is with monthly injections of *hydroxocobalamin* (Neocytamen$_{GB}$) 1000 mg indefinitely. Care must be taken not to inadvertently treat vitamin B_{12} deficiency with folate as this may accelerate the neurological complications.

Folate deficiency results from inadequate intake, malabsorption, increased demand (pregnancy and hyperbolic states) and from certain drugs such as anticonvulsants.

Clinical features are those of anaemia and glossitis. Treatment is with oral *folate* 5 mg twice daily until the underlying cause of the anaemia has been corrected.

Dental significance

In all megaloblastic anaemias, whether of vitamin B_{12} or folate deficiency, atrophic glossitis, angular stomatitis and mouth ulcers are common and may be the presenting symptoms of the condition. The dentist should be alert to the possibility when seeing patients with these signs in the mouth. The oral manifestations of the condition clear up quickly with correction of the deficiency.

Normochromic normocytic anaemias

These anaemias are not due to any deficiency but are the result of associated disease and respond only to correction of the causative disorder. They are seen in the following conditions: chronic infection, e.g. tuberculosis; renal failure; malignancy; liver disease; collagen disorders; endocrine disorders, e.g. myxoedema.

Aplastic anaemia

Aplasia of the bone marrow may be primary where the cause is unknown, or secondary to the toxic action of drugs, chemicals and physical agents. Clinical features are those of anaemia, such as tiredness, increased susceptibility to infection due to the leucopenia, and bleeding resulting from thrombocytopenia. It is commonly fatal; factors influencing prognosis are the aetiology, bleeding problems and infection.

Dental significance

Extensive oral ulceration and haemorrhagic gingivitis may be seen in the mouth as a result of the leucopenia. Extractions should be avoided and only carried out under antibiotic cover, anticipating increased post-extraction haemorrhage. Advice and assistance with oral hygiene is of paramount importance and local analgesics prescribed to ease discomfort (*see* Leukaemia).

Haemolytic anaemias

These result from increased breakdown of red blood cells occurring because of corpuscular defects which include hereditary spherocytosis and hereditary haemaglobinopathies (thalassaemia and sickle-cell disease).

Hereditary spherocytosis

A defect in the red cell leads to its spherocytic shape. It is inherited as a mendelian dominant, presenting with anaemia or jaundice. Complications include pigment gallstones, leg ulcers, splenomegaly, splenic infarction and haemolytic crises. Diagnosis depends on the clinical and haematological features together with the family history. Treatment is by splenectomy.

Thalassaemias

These are a group of inherited disorders due to defective synthesis of the α- and β-chains of haemoglobin.

β-Thalassaemia major presents early in life with anaemia and splenomegaly and, in its severe form, death often occurs in the first year of life. Milder forms are compatible with survival to adulthood.

β-Thalassaemia minor (trait), the heterozygous form, is often symptomless, anaemia is mild and slight splenomegaly occurs. Life expectancy is normal. There is no specific treatment. Occasionally splenectomy is indicated and transfusion necessary.

α-Thalassaemia major causes death of the fetus.

α-Thalassaemia minor, the heterozygous form, is symptomless (high incidence in patients from Cyprus, Greece and northern Italy).

Sickle-cell disease

In this hereditary disorder, the red cells contain HbS, which is less soluble especially in its reduced form leading to deformity of the red cell and the characteristic sickle shape. It occurs most commonly in Negroes of African origin but is seen rarely in certain parts of southern Europe.

Clinical features result from chronic haemolytic anaemia and vascular obstruction due to high viscosity which results in ischaemia and infarction. Sickling crises occur, causing severe pain in bone, joints and, sometimes, abdominal pain with vomiting. Gallstones are common. Central nervous system manifestations result from obstruction of cerebral vessels. Due to repeated splenic infarction the spleen is usually small in adults. Crises are precipitated by infection, stress, exposure to cold, fatigue and anoxia. There is no specific treatment.

Dental significance

Osteomyelitis of the mandible has been reported in those suffering from this condition but the main concern of the dentist lies in a sickling crisis being precipitated by anoxia under a general anaesthetic. The sickling trait can be detected by laboratory examination of the blood or by the dentist in the surgery using a Sickledex. Under ideal conditions all patients of West Indian or African origin should be tested before receiving a general anaesthetic and, if positive, the anaesthetic administered in hospital. In areas with a large immigrant population, this may present practical difficulties. Sickling only occurs with anoxia, and dental anaesthetics are not a hazard if this is remembered and the anaesthetic conducted with 50% oxygen in the anaesthetic gases.

Acquired haemolytic anaemia

This may be acute or chronic, idiopathic or secondary to a variety of causes, virus infection, drugs, underlying disease such as chronic lymphatic leukaemia, lymphomata and systemic lupus erythematosus. It may occur at any age and in 50% of cases is idiopathic.

Acute acquired haemolytic anaemia occurs most commonly in children and runs a short course usually with complete remission.

Chronic acquired haemolytic anaemia occurs mostly in adults and lasts months or years. It is usually associated with antibodies in the blood and is much commoner than the acute form.

Treatment consists of steroids, blood transfusion and sometimes splenectomy. In most cases steroids will induce a remission.

Dental significance

There are no contraindications to routine dentistry but general anaesthetics should be conducted with a high concentration of oxygen in the anaesthetic gases and with special precautions if steroids have been used in treatment (*see* Adrenal insufficiency).

With severe haemolytic anaemias, notably β-thalassaemia, there is hypoplasia of the bone marrow which also affects the bones of the face. In some instances there is swelling of the maxilla on the buccal aspect of the upper teeth giving a 'chipmunk' appearance to the patient.

ANAPHYLAXIS

This is a type I, immediate hypersensitivity reaction in which the allergic agents combined to a protein component interact with IgE antibodies leading to a massive release of vasoactive compounds causing widespread vasodilatation and smooth muscle contraction. Most commonly it is the result of a drug reaction, usually following injection of the drug, but it can occur after oral administration. The risk is greatly enhanced where there has been a previous reaction, often quite mild, such as a maculopapular rash. Initial symptoms are often a generalized pruritus, especially on the soles and palms, hyperaemia of the skin, angio-oedema, resulting in a fall in circulating blood volume, vascular collapse and shock. The patient may experience a metallic taste in the mouth, an urge to micturate or defaecate and sometimes severe bronchospasm. Prolonged unconsciousness or vomiting may occur. Death may result from cardiac arrhythmias or asphyxia.

Prompt treatment is of paramount importance if lives are to be saved. First clear the airway, if the patient has vomited, and administer oxygen. *Adrenaline* 0.5–1.0 ml of 1:1000 should be given intramuscularly and repeated at intervals of 5 minutes, if necessary, to sustain a measurable blood pressure. Subcutaneous adrenaline may not be absorbed fast enough and this route is not advised. In addition *hydrocortisone* 200 mg i.v. and an antihistamine such as *chlorpheniramine* (Piriton injection$_{GB}$) 10 mg i.m. should be given. As soon as resuscitation measures have been commenced, arrangements should be made to transfer the patient to hospital with a dental or medical escort to continue treatment as required. An intravenous line should be established as soon as possible.

Dental significance

Fortunately acute anaphylaxis is a rare sequel of drugs used in the dental surgery. Those more likely to provoke it are *penicillin, barbiturates* and anaesthetic agents. Brief questioning of the patient as to any previous experience is a wise precaution before using these.

ANEURYSM

For aneurysm, *see under* Vascular disease–Arterial aneurysm.

ANGINA PECTORIS

For angina pectoris, *see under* Heart disease, ischaemic.

ANGIO-OEDEMA

In the more common, non-hereditary form of this disease, swelling of the face and mouth can occur as an allergic reaction, although the particular allergen cannot always be traced. The oedema is not dangerous and subsides on its own in a number of days. Antihistamines, such as *chlorpheniramine* (Piriton$_{GB}$) 4 mg four times daily may help. A rare familial form of the disease results from an abnormality of the serum complement system. The oedema, which may involve the glottis, is sometimes provoked by trauma such as dental extractions. Prophylaxis with androgens and antifibrinolytic drugs has proved helpful in those subject to the condition. Treatment of an attack may require intramuscular *adrenaline* (0.5–1 ml of 1:1000), *hydrocortisone* 100 mg i.v., and tracheotomy if the airway is threatened.

Dental significance

In the non-hereditary angio-oedema, the dentist should diligently enquire whether the attack appears to follow dental treatment, the fitting of any appliance or the use of medicaments in the mouth. If so these should be avoided in the future.

Patients suffering from the familial form of the disease will usually be aware of it. Extractions and endodontics should be undertaken in hospital after infusion with fresh plasma.

ANKYLOSING SPONDYLITIS

This is an erosive inflammatory arthropathy affecting the sacroiliac joints and spine with a strong tendency to fixation of the spine. Most commonly it affects young men. There is a familial incidence and a characteristic tissue type HLA-27, indicating a genetic factor. Ulcerative colitis and Crohn's disease are seen more commonly with this condition than in the general population.

Dental significance

Reclining dental chairs have made it easier to treat these patients in the surgery.

Occasionally the temporomandibular joint is involved in the disease and patients are unable to open their mouth more than 0.5 cm. Dental treatment must be adapted to what is possible with the limited access, and the patient helped with advice and mechanical aids to oral hygiene. General anaesthetics are a hazard and should only be administered in hospital.

ANOREXIA NERVOSA

This is a prolonged illness principally of young girls after puberty, characterized by gross weight loss which is self-induced, amenorrhoea and psychological disturbance. The aetiology is unknown. Diagnosis is based on recognizing the clinical features of the illness and excluding organic disease, severe depressive illness or schizophrenia. As the condition progresses hypotension, bradycardia, blue cold peripheries and fine downy hair (lanugo) develop. Physical over-activity is often marked despite severe emaciation. There is no specific treatment but general management is of the greatest importance, the main aim being the correction of the nutritional state and the psychiatric disturbance.

Dental significance

Extension enamel erosion is encountered either as a result of taking acid fruit juice or from purposeful vomiting after eating. It is most noticeable on the palatal surface of the upper incisors.

ANTHRAX

A rare disorder in the UK caused by *Bacillus anthracis* and usually affecting animals. Man may be infected by close contact with diseased animals or their carcasses. The characteristic lesion is a sore with a coal-black centre which may affect any part of the body but is frequently on the face or neck. Less commonly, pulmonary or intestinal involvement may occur.

Treatment is with penicillin, resistance being rare.

Dental significance

A lesion in the mouth has been reported, but is extremely rare.

APLASTIC ANAEMIA

For aplastic anaemia, *see under* Anaemia.

ASPERGILLOSIS

A number of different disease states result from fungi of the genus *Aspergillus*.

Aspergillus species are often isolated from patients with chronic obstructive airways disease but are usually not of clinical significance.

Allergic bronchopulmonary aspergillosis is usually associated with *A. fumigatus*, and tends to occur in predisposed subjects such as atopics. Reversible airway obstruction occurs, but with advanced disease breathlessness and a chronic productive cough occur. Diagnosis is made by a positive aspergillus prick test, eosinophilia and *Aspergillus* sp. in the sputum.

Aspergilloma, a fungal ball, may occur in existing lung cavities, usually causing no symptoms but occasionally causing haemoptysis.

Invasive aspergillosis occurs rarely in immunodeficient individuals (i.e. leukaemia, neutropenia, AIDS and treatment with immunosuppressives). Treatment is with parenteral *amphotericin B*.

Dental significance

Painful haemorrhagic lesions have been described on the tongue and palate but are rare.

ASTHMA

This is a condition of variable breathlessness due to widespread narrowing of peripheral airways which varies in severity over short periods of time, spontaneously or with treatment. The narrowing results from release of various bronchoconstrictor substances in the bronchial wall. Many factors may influence their release: exercise, allergy and infection. Psychological factors and drugs, especially β-adrenergic blockers, may potentiate the effect. Asthma may be divided into:

1. Extrinsic asthma, occurring at a young age with a familial history of allergy, often in atopic subjects, running an intermittent course, associated with raised IgE levels.
2. Intrinsic asthma, occurring in middle age, usually persistent, associated with a family history of asthma, normal levels of IgE and unassociated with atopy.

Treatment

Where possible the allergen is eliminated. Desensitization may be possible. Drug therapy is aimed at treating the acute attack or as a prophylactic measure to prevent attacks.

Treatment of acute attack Sympathomimetic aerosols, *salbutamol* (Ventolin$_{GB}$), *terbutaline* (Bricanyl$_{GB}$, Brethine$_{US}$) or *orciprenaline* (Alupent$_{GB,US}$) are selective, and have a greater effect on the bronchi than the heart.

Prophylactic treatment *Sodium cromoglycate* (Intal$_{GB, US}$) spinhalers or steroid aerosols (*beclomethasone*) are most commonly used for prophylactic treatment. Theophylline derivatives (*aminophylline*) and cholinergic drugs are also of value.
Treatment of a severe attack Treatment involves putting a face mask on the patient and giving oxygen. Next, *hydrocortisone* 200 mg should be given intravenously followed by the slow intravenous injection of *aminophylline* 250 mg in 10 ml of water, given at the rate of 1 ml (25 mg)/minute. Arrangements should be made to transfer the patient to hospital as soon as possible.

Dental significance

There are no contraindications to routine dentistry with local anaesthetics, but patients should be instructed to take the prophylactic measures they have been prescribed and bring with them any aerosol that they use in an attack.

General anaesthetics may be given to those who suffer from mild uncomplicated asthma providing certain precautions are taken. If possible, a time of the year should be chosen when attacks are less frequent. Normal prophylactic treatment should be taken and aerosols brought with the patient. *Atropine* should be given as a premedication (200 μg under 10 years, 400–600 μg over 10 years and adults) either intramuscularly 1 hour before or intravenously at the time of the anaesthetic. If intravenous induction is desired, the amount should be no more than that required to put the patient to sleep and then anaesthesia induced and maintained with 50% oxygen, nitrous oxide and halothane to the concentration required. The drugs required to treat a severe attack of asthma should be readily available.

Aspirin and *aspirin*-containing compounds are best avoided by the chronic asthmatic and the use of non-steroidal anti-inflammatory drugs (NSAIDs), especially *mefenamic acid* (Ponstan$_{GB}$, Ponstel$_{US}$), forbidden.

It is worth remembering that one of the side-effects of nebulized corticosteroids is oropharyngeal candidiasis.

ATHEROMA

For atheroma, *see under* Vascular disease.

AURICULAR FIBRILLATION

For auricular fibrillation, *see* Heart disease, dysrhythmias.

BACTERIAL ENDOCARDITIS

For bacterial endocarditis, *see under* Heart disease, infective – Infective endocarditis.

BEHÇET'S SYNDROME

This condition, seen more frequently in the Mediterranean countries and Japan, is of unknown aetiology. Painful aphthous-type ulcers occur in the mouth and on the genitals together with conjunctivitis or iridocyclitis. A skin eruption, recurrent arthritis affecting arms and legs, and neurological signs may be present. Systemic corticosteroids and immunosuppressive drugs are used to combat the condition but, unlike Reiter's syndrome which it resembles, Behçet's syndrome tends to be chronic and poorly influenced by treatment.

Dental significance

Triamcinolone paste (Adcortyl$_{GB}$, Kenalog$_{US}$) in orobase, or *betamethasone* spray (Betnesol$_{GB}$) to the mouth ulcers four times daily is usually helpful.

BELL'S PALSY

This unilateral facial paralysis is probably due to a localized neuritis of the seventh nerve within the bony canal. The cause remains uncertain, but it is generally thought there may be a viral aetiology and this view is supported by studies that have detected rising antibody titres to a variety of viruses. A similar condition, Ramsay Hunt syndrome, in which the paralysis is accompanied by vesicles round the ear, has been shown to result from herpes zoster of the geniculate ganglion.

The onset is sudden, a patient usually complaining of stiffness in the face when getting up in the morning, and paralysis developing over the next 24–48 hours. Sometimes an alteration in taste is a feature. Recovery starts after a week and is complete for 60–80% of cases, but the prognosis is less favourable for the old and in those in whom the paralysis is total and is associated with severe mastoid pain.

Steroids given as soon as possible after diagnosis offer the best chance of reducing nerve damage. *Prednisolone* 20 mg four times a day should be given for 5 days and then the dosage tailed off over the subsequent 3 weeks.

Dental significance

Because of disfigurement and embarrassment of facial paralysis, a dentist seeing a patient with the early symptoms of Bell's palsy should contact the patient's doctor and, with his blessing, commence treatment with steroids immediately, providing the patient does not suffer from diabetes mellitus or peptic ulceration.

In those with severe paralysis, an acrylic-covered wire hook, set in a part upper denture, may be helpful in holding up the corner of the mouth to prevent dribbling. Food often accumulates in the buccal sulcus and instruction and assistance in oral hygiene is important.

BENIGN MYALGIC ENCEPHALOMYELITIS (BME)

This is also known as Royal Free disease and is an epidemic febrile illness of abrupt onset, characterized by headache, upper respiratory symptoms and fever, associated with fluctuating weakness, paraesthesia, muscle pain and tenderness. Mental symptoms include depression, panic states, amnesia, poor concentration and hallucinations.

Symptoms may be very chronic and relapses are frequent, but no fatal cases have been described.

Treatment is symptomatic, bedrest being important in the acute state followed by a gradual return to activity but avoiding excessive physical exercise. Up to now, the pathogenesis of the condition has remained obscure with no objective evidence of organic nervous disease. However, some recent research has indicated that it may result from viral RNA being transported from the gut to other sites in the body where it interferes with cell function, and a test to confirm diagnosis has been developed.

Dental significance

General anaesthetics are thought to cause adverse reactions and some sufferers appear to be extra sensitive to antibiotics.

BILIARY DISEASE

Cholangitis

Infection of the extrahepatic or intrahepatic biliary tree usually complicates obstruction of the bile ducts due to gallstones, surgery or other causes. The clinical picture is of an acute, often severe, illness characterized by abdominal pain, jaundice, fever and rigors.

Treatment requires high doses of systemic antibiotics, but in the case of biliary obstruction surgical correction of the obstruction may be necessary to control the infection.

Cholecystitis

Inflammation of the gallbladder is frequently, but not always, associated with gallstones. Acute cholecystitis causes abdominal pain, usually over the gallbladder area, tenderness and fever. It is most common in middle-aged women. Complications include perforation, empyema and gangrene of the gallbladder. Treatment is conservative with antibiotics and, provided the patient is responding, with elective surgery at a later date. If the patient is deteriorating urgent surgery may be indicated. Chronic cholecystitis is a poorly understood entity. Flatulent dyspepsia and vague upper abdominal pains are frequently attributed to it, but there is no doubt these symptoms are common in people with normal gallbladders, and cholecystectomy frequently fails to cure the symptoms.

Gallstones

Gallstones result from a disorder of bile secretion in the liver but the stones usually form in the gallbladder rather than the bile ducts. Seventy to eighty per cent of gallstones are asymptomatic. They occur more commonly in women than men, particularly in those who have had children and frequency increases with age. Forty to seventy per cent of women have gallstones by the time they reach old age.

Most gallstones are predominantly cholesterol. Pigment gallstones are seen particularly in the presence of haemolytic blood disorders. The clinical features result from the gallstones obstructing the neck of the gallbladder or common bile duct. The pain is often severe, persistent and frequently related to eating, especially fatty food. An obstructing stone in the gallbladder, which does not pass spontaneously, results in either cholecystitis or a (symptomless) non-functioning gallbladder. Obstruction to the common bile duct causes jaundice, sometimes associated with ascending cholangitis and pancreatitis.

Treatment for symptomatic gallstones is surgical. However, under certain circumstances – for example, where there are strong contraindications to surgery and where the gallstones are radiolucent – dissolution of the gallstones, using *chenodeoxycholic acid* (Chendol$_{GB}$) or *ursodeoxycholic acid* (Destolit$_{GB}$) is sometimes successful.

Dental significance

Jaundice, when present, will be evident in the mucous membrane of the mouth as well as the skin and sclerae of the eyes. With obstructive jaundice there is malabsorption of vitamin K and intramuscular fat-soluble vitamin K, *menadiol sodium phosphate* 10 mg (Synkavit$_{GB}$, Synkayvite$_{US}$) should be given 8 hours prior to any dental extraction.

General anaesthetics should be administered in hospital and halothane avoided as an anaesthetic agent.

BORNHOLM'S DISEASE (EPIDEMIC MYALGIA, PLEURODYNIA)

This condition is caused by Coxsackie virus of the B group. The incubation period is 2–14 days and symptoms develop suddenly with headache, fever and severe pain in the lower chest, abdomen and sometimes limbs. The acute phase usually passes in 2–3 days but fever and less severe pains may last for a week. There is no specific treatment and prognosis is good.

Dental significance

There is no dental significance.

BOWEN'S DISEASE

This is a skin condition of the elderly which takes the form of an asymptomatic raised red plaque with moderate scaling, appearing on the head, neck, trunk or distal limbs. Although it frequently remains stable for some time, squamous cell carcinoma with bleeding and ulceration is apt to develop. In about a fifth of cases there is coexisting internal malignancy.

Treatment is by excision or cryotherapy.

Dental significance

Frequently the lesion is not reported to the patient's doctor and, if on the face, may be first noticed by the patient's dentist. In such a case the patient should be advised to seek medical treatment.

BRONCHIECTASIS

In this condition there is irreversible dilatation of the bronchi, most commonly secondary to infection and obstruction. It usually develops in childhood. It may be localized or widespread and bilateral. Symptoms are of a cough productive of large volumes of purulent sputum. Often the patient remains well with little incapacity. Physical signs include finger clubbing and coarse crepitations in the areas affected. Haemoptysis is a common feature. Complications include pneumonia and rarely pericarditis, cerebral abscess and amyloid.

Treatment consists of teaching the patient effective postural drainage and the use of antibiotics, either in exacerbations of the disease or on a long-term basis. For localized disease surgery may be successful. Prognosis in general is good.

Dental significance

There is no dental significance, unless associated with impaired ventilatory capacity (*see* Bronchitis) or secondary amyloid (*see* Amyloidosis).

BRONCHITIS, CHRONIC

The symptoms of chronic bronchitis result from excessive production of bronchial secretions giving rise to a productive cough on most days for at least 3 months in the year. Because it is frequently associated with airway obstruction, variable degrees of emphysema are common. Chronic bronchitis is closely associated with smoking, working in dusty conditions, poor social circumstances and an urban environment. Initial symptoms consist only of a productive cough but, as the condition progresses, increasing dyspnoea occurs, leading to progressive respiratory failure. In a proportion of patients, right-sided heart failure occurs (cor pulmonale).

Management

Patients who smoke should stop and, where possible, avoid dusty environments. Antibiotics should be used for exacerbations but not on a long-term basis. Where there is significant airway obstruction, bronchodilators should be used and in the more resistant patients steroids may be very beneficial. Complications include pneumonia, pneumothorax, polycythaemia, cor pulmonale and respiratory failure.

Dental significance

General anaesthetics in patients suffering from chronic bronchitis are a hazard. Many bronchitics exist with a raised level of carbon dioxide in the blood and reduced oxygen tension. When this is altered through breathing anaesthetic gases containing higher levels of oxygen and no carbon dioxide, stimulation to breathe ceases. Any patient whose bronchitis is such as to require medical treatment should be referred for an anaesthetic assessment before a general anaesthetic is administered.

BRUCELLOSIS (UNDULANT FEVER)

This is primarily an animal disease, with man becoming an accidental host, either through contact with infected animals or by consumption of infected milk, cream or cheese.

The disease is caused by the bacterium *Brucella* sp. of which there are three species: *B. abortus* mainly in cattle, *B. melitensis* in goat and sheep and *B. suis* in swine. *Brucella* can invade via the gastrointestinal tract, skin, respiratory tract or conjunctiva. The incubation period may be from 2 weeks to many months. The disease may be acute with rigors, sweats, fever, headache and depression. However, the severity of symptoms varies and the illness may be no more than a mild 'flu-like illness.

In the chronic form there may be no acute phase and symptoms include depression, headaches, weakness, sweating, backache, anorexia and insomnia. Diagnosis is confirmed by culturing the organism from a blood sample in the acute phase of the illness, or serological tests.

Treatment in the acute phase is very effective, *tetracycline* (250–500 mg 6-hourly) being the drug of choice. In the chronic form treatment may have little or no effect.

Dental significance

Stomatitis, with numerous small ulcers and oedematous gingivae, has been reported but is not common.

BULIMIA NERVOSA

In this condition, closely related to anorexia nervosa, the patient indulges in periodic 'binge eating' followed by induced vomiting. It is a disease of adolescents and young adults, females being afflicted 10 times more commonly than males. It is generally considered to be a behavioural anomaly, but a raised serum amylase level has been reported in a significant percentage of victims. Profound hypokalaemia may occur.

Dental significance

The condition is seldom reported by the patient, but the observation of enamel erosion on the palatal surface of the teeth should alert the dentist to its presence. Other signs sometimes encountered are swelling of the salivary glands, enlarged masseters and callouses on the dorsum of fingers. As it may progress to the much more dangerous condition of anorexia nervosa, sufferers should be advised to seek medical help.

BURKITT'S LYMPHOMA

For Burkitt's lymphoma, *see under* Lymphoproliferative disease.

C

C

CANDIDA INFECTION (THRUSH)

Infection with the fungus *Candida albicans* can be localized to the mouth, may be acute or chronic or spread widely over the body. The severe form, characterized by large white patches on the tongue, buccal mucosa and elsewhere, is usually associated with immunodeficiency disease, debility, diabetes, malignancy, iron deficiency or prolonged treatment with antibiotics, corticosteroids or cytotoxic drugs. Candida infection of the mouth is the commonest oral manifestation of AIDS and is present in the vast majority of cases. A chronic atrophic form, unrelated to debility or immunodeficiency, is sometimes seen under upper dentures and removable orthodontic appliances.

Chronic mucocutaneous candidiasis is always associated with an immunological defect and is seen in different forms in the young and the elderly.

Treatment must be aimed first at correcting the predisposing factors, general or local. Severe infections require systemic treatment but, if mild and localized to the mouth, topical applications of fungicide held in the mouth for several minutes four times daily will be effective. Preparations include *nystatin* (Nystan oral suspension$_{GB}$, Mycostatin$_{US}$), *amphotericin* lozenges (Fungilin$_{GB}$) and *miconazole* (Daktarin oral gel$_{GB}$). Infections of the skin should be treated with 1% *clotrimazole* cream (Canestan$_{GB}$, Mycelex$_{US}$, Lotrimin$_{US}$). *Ketoconazole* (Nizoral$_{GB}$) 400 mg daily is a systemic fungicide given by mouth for severe infections. It depends on stomach acid for utilization and so is ineffective in patients on alkalis or H_2-receptor antagonists. It can be hepatotoxic and liver function tests are required after 10 days' use.

Dental significance

The diagnosis of acute oral thrush is usually obvious but can be confirmed by scraping off one of the white patches which will show the typical hyphae when examined microscopically. The chronic form seen under an appliance must be distinguished fom allergy to the appliance material. The denture or applicance should be left out at night, and it is usually advised that it be left soaking in 0.2% *chlorhexidine* solution and coated with a fungicidal gel (Nystangel$_{GB}$, Mycostatin$_{US}$ oral suspension).

Candida leukoplakia appearing in the floor of the mouth or on the sides of the tongue must be considered as precancerous (*see* Leukoplakia).

CARCINOID SYNDROME

This condition is characterized by flushing, diarrhoea, wheezing and cardiac disease and is due to secretion of various vasoactive substances, 5-hydroxytryptamine, bradykinin and histamine, by carcinoid tumour tissue. These tumours arise from the argentaffin cells of the gut and are most frequently found in the ileum. The syndrome only occurs once the tumour has metastasized to the liver, and thus the prognosis for the syndrome is usually poor. The most common symptom is flushing which is paroxysmal but may be precipitated by certain foods, alcohol and excitement. Diarrhoea is variable and not always present. Like the flushing, asthma is paroxysmal and usually accompanies the flushing when present. In carcinoid heart disease, the right side of the heart is more commonly affected. Fibrous tissue is laid down on the endothelium of the heart causing pulmonary stenosis and tricuspid incompetence. Diagnosis is confirmed by measuring the metabolite 5-hydroxyindole acetic acid in the urine. Treatment is mainly symptomatic; rarely is surgery indicated or of benefit.

Dental significance

As stated, the prognosis in this condition is poor though patients may survive for several years. Dentistry must be planned with this in mind. By reason of the cardiac and bronchial complication, general anaesthetics should be avoided and, if essential, administered in hospital.

CARDIAC ARREST

For cardiac arrest, *see under* Heart disease, ischaemic.

CHICKENPOX

For chickenpox, *see* Varicella.

CHOLANGITIS

For cholangitis, *see under* Biliary disease.

CHOLECYSTITIS

For cholecystitis, *see under* Biliary disease.

CHOREA

Huntington's disease

This disease is inherited as a mendelian dominant, although sporadic cases occur. It appears between the ages of 30 and 45 and progresses from choreiform movements to dementia and complete incapacity. The duration of the disease is 5–30 years. The cause is unknown. There is no treatment other than sedation.

Dental significance

If dental procedures have to be performed, a general anaesthetic will be necessary, because only then will the athetoid movements cease.

Sydenham's chorea (St Vitus' dance)

This is a condition characterized by complex involuntary movements which are variable and may involve several muscles. The cause is unknown but is thought to be rheumatic inflammation of the brain in view of its association with acute rheumatism and rheumatic heart disease. It is now rare but was common 25 years ago. It occurs between the ages of 5 and 15, often associated with emotional instability. Recovery occurs in 6 weeks to 3 months.

Treatment is by complete bedrest and careful nursing. *Salicylates* are of value and sedation may be beneficial.

Dental significance

A medical history of Sydenham's chorea will alert the dentist to the likelihood of valvular disease of the heart. Antibiotic cover will be required for dental procedures likely to cause a bacteraemia (*see* Heart disease, infective—Infective endocarditis). General anaesthetics should not be given without an assessment by a physician.

CHRISTMAS DISEASE

For Christmas disease, *see* Haemophilia, Christmas disease and von Willebrand's disease.

CIRRHOSIS

For cirrhosis, *see under* Liver disease.

COARCTATION OF THE AORTA

For coarctation of the aorta, *see under* Heart disease, congenital.

COELIAC DISEASE

One in 2000 of the general population suffers with coeliac disease in the UK, and it constitutes the commonest cause of malabsorption. More than one member of a family may have the condition which is associated with the skin condition, dermatitis herpetiformis and the tissue type HLA-B8. The basic defect is due to a poorly understood interaction between a fraction of gluten (α-gliaden) and the small intestinal mucosa. This results in damage and flattening of the mucosal villi. The clinical consequences of this 'flat' mucosa are diarrhoea and weight loss together with other features of malabsorption such as anaemia and osteomalacia. Mouth ulceration is an unexplained associated finding. The condition may present in infancy with diarrhoea and failure to thrive, or for the first time in adult life. Diarrhoea may be absent, making diagnosis difficult and delayed.

Once suspected, the diagnosis is confirmed with a jejunal biopsy and by observing improvement on a gluten-free diet. Such a diet leads to complete recovery; however, gluten is contained in all cereal crops and all food products made from them have to be constituted from specially prepared flour.

Untreated, the disease may lead to severe malnutrition and death, a serious but rare complication being small bowel lymphoma.

Dental significance

Recurrent aphthous ulcers are seen in about a quarter of patients with this disease. They clear up with treatment of the primary condition but resolution may be assisted by topical steroids in the form of *hydrocortisone* lozenges (Corlan_{GB}) 2.5 mg or *triamcinolone* paste (Adcortyl_{GB}, Kenalog_{US}) in orobase.

Enamel hypoplasia is found when the disease has been present since infancy and the signs of osteomalacia when it has remained untreated.

Anaemia is a common complication and must be borne in mind if general anaesthetics are required.

COLITIS

The term means inflammation of the colon. The main causes are, for specific colitis: pseudomembranous colitis, ischaemic colitis, radiation colitis and infective colitis (amoebic and tuberculous); and for non-specific colitis: ulcerative colitis and Crohn's colitis.

Pseudomembranous colitis

This condition presents with typical colitic symptoms, rectal bleeding, diarrhoea and abdominal pain. It is most commonly the result of antibiotics, particularly *clindamycin* (Dalacin C_{GB}, $Cleocin_{US}$) and *lincomycin* ($Lincocin_{GB,US}$) although it has now been reported following almost all antibiotics. It results from the effects of a toxin produced by the bacterium *Clostridium difficile.* This can be isolated from the stools and the toxin can be identified. In the florid form of the disease the large bowel mucosa has a characteristic appearance, being partly covered by white plaques which when removed leave a bleeding area of mucosa. The condition can vary from a mild diarrhoeal illness to severe total colitis, sometimes requiring colectomy. There is unfortunately no way of predicting who is liable to develop this complication of antibiotic therapy, and the worrying fact is that it can develop following only very limited courses of antibiotics.

Treatment is symptomatic. Specific treatment is with *vancomycin* or *metronidazole*.

Ischaemic colitis

This condition is most commonly seen in the elderly and results from arteriosclerotic disease of the mesenteric vessels. It may present acutely with bloody diarrhoea which may progress to gut infarction, or it may present with diarrhoea associated with ischaemic stricture formation. Treatment is symptomatic.

Ulcerative colitis

This inflammatory disease of the colon is of unknown aetiology and more common in the second to fourth decades. In the West its prevalence is 5 per 100 000. The severity of the condition varies from a mild intermittent diarrhoeal illness to a life-threatening disease. The direct complications include toxic dilatation of the colon, perforation, massive bleeding and carcinoma, while indirect complications are uveitis, iritis, erythema nodosum, arthritis and cirrhosis.

Treatment consists of symptomatic treatment of the diarrhoea with *codeine phosphate, diphenoxylate* ($Lomotil_{GB}$), or *loperamide hydrochloride* (Imodium$_{GB, US}$) and anti-inflammatory treatment with *sulphasalazine* (Salazopyrin$_{GB}$, Azulfidine$_{US}$) and *prednisolone* given either systemically or topically in the form of enemas or suppositories. Some people are unable to tolerate *sulphasalazine* because of side-effects – skin rashes, nausea or headaches. A new preparation, *mersalazine* (Asacol$_{GB}$), the 5-aminosalicyclic acid component of the *salazopyrine* molecule, has recently been released to counter this problem. Surgery (colectomy) is curative but almost invariably results in a permanent ileostomy.

Dental significance

Recurrent aphthous ulceration of the mouth is not uncommon in patients with ulcerative colitis. Its severity corresponds to that of the bowel condition and improves with medical or surgical treatment of the primary disease. Topical steroids in the form of *hydrocortisone* pellets (Corlan$_{GB}$) or *triamcinolone* paste (Adcortyl$_{GB}$, Kenalog$_{US}$) in orobase, are helpful. If discomfort is severe a viscous mouthwash containing 2% *lignocaine* will make eating less of a misery. Dentists must appreciate that most cases of pseudomembranous colitis are the direct result of treatment with antibiotics, especially *clindamycin* (Dalacin C$_{GB}$, Cleocin$_{US}$) and *lincomycin* (Lincocin$_{GB, US}$). No antibiotic should be prescribed without good cause, and these two only for infections where the organism is insensitive to safer alternatives.

Patients under treatment with *diphenoxylate* and *atropine* (Lomotil$_{GB}$) may suffer from xerostomia and conscientious attention to oral hygiene and caries control is most important. Those receiving *prednisolone* systemically or rectally must be treated as cases of adrenal insufficiency and appropriate precautions taken (*see* Adrenal insufficiency). Research has shown NSAIDs to be a factor in the relapse of treated cases of ulcerative colitis, and they should be used with extreme caution in patients with a history of the condition.

CONN'S SYNDROME

For Conn's syndrome, *see under* Adrenal disease.

CORONARY THROMBOSIS

For coronary thrombosis, *see under* Heart disease, ischaemic.

COR PULMONALE

This is a right-sided heart failure secondary to obstruction in the pulmonary circulation or more commonly chronic lung disease.

Dental significance

General anaesthetics are to be avoided.

COXIELLA BURNETTI (Q FEVER)

This is a rickettsial disease due to the organism *Coxiella burnetti*. The disease is mild and characterized by pneumonitis, but occasionally gives rise to hepatitis or endocarditis. Treatment is with *chloramphenicol* or *tetracycline*.

Dental significance

There is no dental significance.

CRANIAL ARTERITIS

For cranial arteritis, *see under* Giant cell arteritis.

CRETINISM

For cretinism, *see* Thyroid disease.

CROHN'S DISEASE

This inflammatory bowel disease of unknown aetiology occurs most commonly between the second and fourth decade and appears to be increasing in incidence. Any part of the bowel may be affected from mouth to anus, the distribution being characteristically patchy and the full thickness of the bowel being involved.

Presentation is extremely variable, abdominal pain and diarrhoea being the commonest symptoms but anorexia, weight loss, fever, night sweats, vomiting and anaemia may all occur as presenting features with or without diarrhoea.

Diagnosis is based on radiological and histological appearances.

In addition to symptomatic treatment for pain and diarrhoea, replacement therapy is required for nutritional deficiencies and specific anti-inflammatory treatment for control of the disease. The choice of drug is extremely limited. *Prednisolone* is the only generally effective medical treatment, the dose being varied between 5 and 60 mg/day depending on the severity of the disease. *Sulphasalazine* (Salazopyrin$_{GB}$, Azulfidine$_{US}$) 2–4 g/day may be beneficial in colonic but not small bowel Crohn's disease. Immunosuppressive therapy is of no proven value.

Remissions and relapses are the pattern of the disease. There is no known cure. Surgery when necessary is conservative, in view of the recurrent nature of the disease. Complications are similar to those seen in ulcerative colitis.

Dental significance

Oral ulceration, varying from mild aphthous to deep indurated ulcers, is seen in some 10% of patients suffering from Crohn's disease. Areas of the mucous membrane of the mouth may show granulomatous infiltration similar to that found in the small intestine. Topical steroid treatment with *hydrocortisone* pellets (Corlan$_{GB}$) or *triamcinolone* paste (Adcortyl$_{GB}$, Kenalog$_{US}$) in orobase, is usually effective and 0.2% *chlorhexidine* (Corsodyl$_{GB}$, Peridex$_{US}$) as a mouthwash used four times a day will prevent secondary infection. If discomfort is severe a viscous mouthwash containing 2% *lignocaine* will make eating less of a misery.

CRYPTOCOCCOSIS

This is a systemic yeast infection caused by *Cryptococcus neoformans*, most commonly causing meningitis but also involving the lungs and skin. A disseminated form is also recognized. The yeast is most commonly found in pigeon droppings. It may particularly infect immunocomprised individuals.

Dental significance

In those with suppressed immunity, granulomatous lesions may be present in the mouth.

CUSHING'S DISEASE

For Cushing's disease, *see under* Adrenal disease.

CYSTIC FIBROSIS (FIBROCYSTIC DISEASE, MUCOVISCIDOSIS)

This condition is due to a defect of cell membrane function resulting in diminished sodium reabsorption. Body secretions are abnormal in either viscosity or volume. There are three main clinical manifestations of this inherited defect:

1. Meconium ileus: the viscid mucus results in solidification of intestinal contents in the neonate with intestinal obstruction. The prognosis is extremely poor.
2. Gastrointestinal: chronic diarrhoea and steatorrhoea occur due to pancreatic insufficiency resulting from obstruction to pancreatic ducts by viscous secretions.
3. Respiratory: recurrent infections lead to bronchiectasis and emphysema. If untreated, 80% die in the first year of life, usually from bronchopneumonia. With prompt treatment of superadded infections 75% may reach adolescence. However, mean survival in the best centres is only 12 years. *Pseudomonas* sp. is often the infective organism and *ceftazidime* ($\text{Fortum}_{\text{GB}}$), and more recently *ciprofloxacin* ($\text{Ciproxin}_{\text{GB}}$), are the drugs of choice for treatment.

The disease is genetic and apparently transmitted by an autosomal recessive trait. Screening is now possible and, when both parents are shown to be carriers, advice should be given to them about having children.

Dental significance

Chronic sinusitis is a feature of the condition and enlargement of the submandibular salivary glands has been reported. General anaesthetics should only be administered in hospital.

CYTOMEGALOVIRUS INFECTION

The condition may result from spontaneous infection or can be spread by transfused blood. It is frequently associated with AIDS and other states of suppressed immunity. Although often symptomless, it may be associated with a sore throat and lymphadenopathy, and more rarely the manifestations of encephalitis, pneumonitis, myopericarditis, hepatitis or thrombocytopenia and anaemia. A mononucleosis is usual but the heterophile antibody test is negative. The virus can be cultured from body fluids and the pharynx.

The main worry about the infection is that it is transmitted to the fetus *in utero* and produces congenital defects.

There is no specific treatment and *acyclovir* (Zovirax$_{GB,US}$) is only weakly effective.

Dental significance

It would seem logical that infection could be spread via the dental surgery, but provided instruments and equipment are sterilized by autoclave or viricidal agents, the danger must be remote. If suspected, nursing staff who might be pregnant should not assist at treatment.

DEMENTIA

For dementia, *see* Alzheimer's disease and Psychiatric disorders.

DERMATOMYOSITIS

This is a collagen disorder characterized by diffuse inflammation of skin and muscle, the cause of which is unknown. Women are affected twice as often as men, and the peak age is between 30 and 50. In 15% of adults, there is an associated underlying carcinoma.

The symptoms are malaise, myalgia, weakness and fatigue. The rash occurs over the V of the neck and extensor surfaces of the limbs. Erythema can affect the face giving a typical heliotrope colour with periorbital oedema.

Diagnosis is clinical and may be confirmed by muscle biopsy.

Steroids are the mainstay of medical treatment. Surgery may be indicated for underlying malignancy and can lead to symptomatic improvement. In general prognosis is poor, 50% of patients dying in 3 years.

Dental significance

In a number of cases, oedema of the mucous membranes and a red–blue erythema is found in the mouth. Steroid treatment must be taken into consideration if extractions are contemplated (*see* Adrenal insufficiency). General anaesthetics should be administered in hospital.

DIABETES INSIPIDUS

This condition results from deficient production of antidiuretic hormone due to disease or damage to the hypothalamus or posterior pituitary. The symptoms of polyuria and polydipsia may rapidly lead to severe dehydration if fluid losses cannot be replaced.

Treatment involves correction of the underlying cause where possible and replacement therapy with *antidiuretic hormone* (Lypressin$_{GB}$, Pitressin$_{US}$) administered as a nasal spray or in more severe cases as an intramuscular injection.

Dental significance

In the untreated disease a dry mouth, with the associated problems of xerostomia, will be a feature.

DIABETES MELLITUS

This is a clinical syndrome caused by the disturbance of carbohydrate, fat and protein metabolism resulting from a deficiency of insulin. It is common, 12–14% of adults having an abnormal glucose tolerance curve. There are approximately 400 000 people with clinical diabetes in England and Wales at the present time.

The aetiology is not clear, but there is an inherited tendency to diabetes and a close correlation with obesity.

Diabetes may be latent and brought on by stress, asymptomatic with abnormal biochemistry only or symptomatic. The majority of diabetics fall into one of two groups:

1. The juvenile type in which those afflicted are typically young, thin, ketotic, insulin dependent, and the diabetes insulin sensitive.
2. The maturity-onset type in which the diabetics tend to be obese, non-ketotic, have mild symptoms, are often not insulin dependent and the condition is insulin resistant.

The clinical presentation may be very variable. The insulin-dependent diabetic may present acutely with the classic features of diabetic ketoacidosis, severe thirst, polyuria, loss of weight, vomiting and anorexia. On examination the patient is dehydrated, overbreathing, drowsy, occasionally comatose and with a smell of ketones on the breath. By contrast, diabetes may be a chance finding complicating other diseases, or may present with the complications of the disease itself.

Diagnosis depends on the glucose tolerance test with a 2-hour blood glucose level greater than 10 mmol/l.

Being a multisystem disease, complications can be multiple and varied. Vision may be impaired due to cataract formation and diabetic retinopathy. Renal function may be affected due either to the increased tendency to renal infection or to intrinsic renal damage leading to glomerulosclerosis and renal failure (Kimmelstiel–Wilson kidney). Infections generally are more common. Atherosclerosis involves both large and small arteries leading to an increased risk of cerebral and cardiovascular complications, and skin ulceration associated with small-vessel involvement. The nervous system can be affected either centrally or peripherally, giving rise to acute and chronic peripheral neuropathy, autonomic neuropathy, diabetic amyotrophy, neuropathic ulceration, impotence and diarrhoea.

Treatment may be subdivided into diet, oral hypoglycaemic agents, insulin and emergency treatment.

Diet

Obese elderly patients with no ketosis may be managed with a low-carbohydrate diet.

Oral hypoglycaemic agents

In non-ketotic patients, where diet does not suffice to control the blood sugar, oral hypoglycaemic agents may be used. There are two types:

1. Sulphonylureas which augment insulin secretion:
   (*a*) *tolbutamide* (Rastinon_{GB}, Orinase_{US}) – a short-acting agent;
   (*b*) *chlorpropamide* ($\text{Diabinese}_{GB, US}$) – a long-acting agent;
   (*c*) *glibenclamide* (Daonil_{GB}) – an intermediate-acting agent.
2. Biguanides, e.g. *metformin* (Glucophage_{GB}) which inhibit glucose absorption from the gut and glucose oxidation.

Insulin

Underweight patients with ketosis should always be treated with insulin, of which there are three main types: short, intermediate and long-acting. Short-acting insulin is soluble and of rapid onset; *isophane* and *insulin zinc* suspension are intermediate-acting insulins and Ultratard is a slow-onset and long-acting insulin. Most patients can be managed best by starting on a twice daily dose of intermediate-acting insulin with short-acting insulin added to cover hyperglycaemia related to breakfast or the evening meal.

Human insulin which has a different amino acid sequence from animal insulin has recently become available and, in theory, should be less immunogenic. However, this appears not to be the case in practice and human and highly purified animal insulins are comparable in action.

Emergency treatment of diabetic ketosis and coma

Treatment of these emergency situations requires hospital admission. The main aspects of treatment are rehydration, administration of soluble insulin, correction of acid–base imbalance and management of complications.

Hypoglycaemia and hypoglycaemic coma

These result from excessive therapy with oral agents and insulin, or normal therapy in the presence of inadequate calorie intake.

Symptoms are hunger, faintness, sweating and aggressiveness progressing to coma. Treatment is with oral *glucose* in the cooperative conscious patient and intravenous *dextrose* (50 ml of 50% *dextrose*) in the presence of pre-coma or coma. Alternatively glucagon 1 mg can be given and has the advantage that it can be injected by any route.

If treated, hypoglycaemic coma does not carry the serious consequences of hyperglycaemic coma and admission to hospital may not be necessary. Delay in treatment can lead to irreversible brain damage.

Dental significance

Because oral manifestations may be among the first, the dentist often plays an important part in the diagnosis of this disease or in warning sufferers when blood sugar control is inadequate. Xerostomia, associated with a bad taste and a burning tongue, is a frequent complaint. Candida patches, periodontal disease and an unexplained increase in caries are other features. Bell's palsy is more common in diabetics.

Scrupulous oral hygiene is important. Routine dental treatment in controlled diabetics can be carried out without special precautions. However, it should be appreciated that infection and stress will increase the patient's demand for *insulin*. Extractions and surgery under local anaesthesia are permissible in general dental practice provided the patient's meal routine is not going to be disturbed for more than a few hours afterwards. General anaesthetics for simple extractions may be given to those patients whose diabetes is controlled by diet alone, provided there is no sepsis or history of coronary occlusion. The morning dose of hypoglycaemic is best omitted to compensate for pre-anaesthetic fasting (hyperglycaemia is safer than hypoglycaemia). Patients who require *insulin* to control their condition should only receive general anaesthetics in hospital where their blood sugar can be monitored.

Aspirin can enhance the effect of oral hypoglycaemic agents, if taken in quantity. Alternative analgesics should be prescribed to relieve dental pain in diabetic patients being treated with these drugs.

Hypo- *vs* hyperglycaemic coma

The dental practitioner may be worried about the distinction between hyper- and hypoglycaemic coma. In practice this problem is unlikely to arise and is not difficult to resolve if it does. Hyperglycaemic coma develops gradually in a patient who is clearly ill and unlikely to be visiting his dentist. As infection is the commonest precipitating factor, the patient is usually toxic and febrile with a hot dry skin and ketotic breath. Hypoglycaemia usually results from inappropriate *insulin* dosage and develops rapidly, usually in a patient who has been quite well up until the time of the coma. Prodromal symptoms are faintness, sweating, hunger and aggressiveness. The comatose patient is not febrile or ketotic. If in doubt intravenous *glucose* therapy will rapidly resolve the problem, rousing the patient with hypoglycaemia and having no effect on the patient with hyperglycaemia who needs to be transferred urgently to hospital.

DIVERTICULAR DISEASE

This term is most commonly applied to the presence of diverticula in the colon. These are herniations of the mucous membrane through the muscle wall of the gut. They may occur throughout the colon but are usually found in the sigmoid region. The condition is extremely common in Western society, 30% of the population over 60 years of age being affected.

Symptoms consist of abdominal pain and alteration in bowel habit, but in the majority of cases the condition is symptomless.

Complications include bleeding, inflammation and abscess formation (diverticulitis).

Dental significance

There is no dental significance.

DIVERTICULITIS

For diverticulitis, *see above under* Diverticular disease.

DOWN'S SYNDROME

The condition results from chromosome imbalance and has a frequency of 1 in 650 live births. It is more common in children of older mothers.

There is mental handicap of a variable degree and impaired resistance to infections. Cardiac and skeletal defects are not uncommon and the incidence of diabetes, hypothyroidism and leukaemia is increased. There is no treatment, but children brought up in the home overcome their difficulties better than those in institutions.

Dental significance

A large fissured tongue, an open bite and a class III malocclusion are the usual presenting features. Delayed eruption with missing or malformed teeth is frequent. Liability to caries is not increased, but periodontal disease and ulcerative gingivitis are common problems.

Generally, the children are cooperative and, with careful handling, routine dental treatment can be undertaken.

A mouth-gag may help a child to keep his mouth open and be a precaution against being bitten. Local anaesthetics should be used where required and sedation may be helpful, although unpredictable. The importance of oral hygiene should be stressed.

Antibiotic cover (*penicillin V* or *amoxycillin* 250 mg three times daily) is advised for extractions, while general anaesthetics should be approached with care because of the possibility of cardiac abnormalities. In 2–3% of cases, there is instability of the atlantoaxial joint and pressure can be put on the spinal cord during a general anaesthetic. Down's syndrome patients cared for in institutions are more likely to be carriers of hepatitis B, and should be treated as high-risk cases in this respect.

DUODENAL ULCER

For duodenal ulcer, *see* Peptic ulceration.

DYSTROPHIA MYOTONICA

This is a hereditary disorder appearing between the ages of 20 and 30 and characterized by myotonia and muscle wasting. The wasting is seen in the facial muscles, sternomastoids, shoulder girdle, forearms, quadriceps and leg muscles. In addition cataracts, frontal balding, dementia and, in men, gonadal atrophy and impotence occur. In women amenorrhoea is usual.

Dental significance

General anaesthetics should be avoided and, if essential, administered in hospital.

EATON–LAMBERT SYNDROME

For Eaton–Lambert syndrome, *see* Myasthenic syndrome.

ECZEMA

Eczema is a reaction of the skin in response to some damaging stimulus which may not be identifiable. Atopic eczema is usually seen in young children, starting on the face and spreading to antecubital and popliteal areas. It is frequently associated with asthma. Subacute and chronic eczema may result from direct skin irritation with chemicals, detergents, cosmetics, or from allergy to drugs or topical medicaments. It is frequently influenced by psychological factors. Infection may complicate it.

Attempts should be made to discover and avoid the precipitating agent. Treatment includes the use of emollients, antimicrobials, antihistamines and corticosteroids.

Dental significance

If systemic *cortisone* has been used in the treatment of the condition, this must be taken into account if oral surgery or general anaesthetics are planned (*see* Adrenal insufficiency).

Dentists and their assistants should try and avoid unnecessary skin contact with medicaments and materials used in their profession.

EHLERS–DANLOS SYNDROME

This condition results from an abnormality of collagen in connective tissue. The skin and mucous membranes are more fragile than normal, and damage and haemorrhage occur with minimal trauma. The teeth are frequently deformed with stunted roots and multiple pulp-stones. Periodontal disease is common.

Dental significance

A gentle touch is essential when working on these patients. Though there is no clotting defect, increased haemorrhage must be expected after extractions, which may be difficult due to tooth fragility. Sutures do not hold adequately in the gingiva. Recurrent dislocation of the temporomandibular joint has been reported.

Orthodontic treatment is not prohibited, but traumatic gingival ulceration from appliances has to be expected and every precaution taken to reduce it to a minimum.

EMBOLISM

This is the blockage of a blood vessel by a clot or collection of abnormal material within the vascular compartment, which has been carried to that site by the blood stream.

Fat emboli may complicate fractures and orthopaedic procedures.

Air emboli occur following trauma or surgical and medical procedures involving large vessels.

Pulmonary emboli

By far the commonest type of embolus is a blood clot and the commonest sites of origin are the deep leg veins or pelvic veins. The clot embolizes to the lungs and may cause immediate fatal obstruction to the pulmonary arterial system. More commonly emboli present with pleuritic pain and haemoptysis. They are seen most commonly in ill, immobile people and constitute a major postoperative complication. An association has been recognized between the contraceptive pill and pulmonary emboli in otherwise fit young women.

Massive pulmonary emboli are usually fatal before treatment is possible. Occasionally surgical intervention is possible. For the majority of patients treatment is by anticoagulation, initially with *heparin* followed by *warfarin*. This treatment is usually continued for some months and sometimes indefinitely where the risk factor persists.

Arterial emboli

These are usually small clots arising in the systemic circulation which occlude arteries of variable size depending on the size of the embolus. They may arise from abnormalities of the left atrium, heart valves and endocardium, or from the walls of the larger arteries. They are seen in association with rheumatic valvular heart disease, infective endocarditis, ischaemic heart disease and atrial fibrillation.

The major organs affected are the brain, gastrointestinal tract, kidneys and limbs. Emboli may cause transient symptoms with no permanent deficit or result in infarction of the tissue supplied by the occluded artery.

Treatment is aimed at preventing further emboli where applicable, removal of the embolus and management of the complications. Anticoagulation may be indicated in certain circumstances.

Dental significance

Oral anticoagulants, such as *warfarin* (Marevan$_{GB}$, Coumadin$_{US}$) prolong the clotting time by antagonism to vitamin K. Their action is potentiated by a number of hypnotics, analgesics, and antibiotics such as *barbiturates, salicylates, chloramphenicol* (Chloromycetin$_{GB,US}$ and Kemicetine $_{GB}$) and *metronidazole* (Flagyl$_{GB,US}$). These should be used with caution on patients being treated with anticoagulants. If extractions are contemplated, the patient's doctor should be consulted with regard to stopping treatment for a few days. Parenteral vitamin K, *menadiol sodium phosphate* (Synkavit$_{GB,US}$) in doses of 10 mg or more will reverse the action of anticoagulants in 24 hours.

EMPHYSEMA

There are two main types of emphysema: pan-acinar and centrilobular.

Pan-acinar

This is dilatation or destruction of the acini.

Centrilobular

This is more proximal dilatation or destruction, involving the respiratory bronchioles.

Aetiology

Emphysema most commonly occurs with long-standing disease of the bronchi, bronchitis, asthma, or a combination of these conditions. It may relate to occupational exposure to dusts. Occasionally it develops as a primary disease.

The major symptom is dyspnoea, increasing with severity of the disease. Progression of symptoms is slow, taking years rather than months. Typically the patient with predominant emphysema is greatly distressed by shortness of breath while remaining pink ('pink puffer'). In contrast, the chronic bronchitic is less troubled by breathlessness though often deeply cyanosed ('blue bloater'). Usually the two conditions coexist and symptoms of both are seen. In established disease, the chest is over-inflated and chest expansion diminished.

Treatment consists of avoidance of harmful environmental factors such as smoke and dust, improvement of the airway by treating any bronchospasm and prompt treatment of superadded infection. Respiratory exercises are valuable, enabling maximum use to be made of the remaining functional lung. The major complications are respiratory failure and right heart failure, cor pulmonale.

Dental significance

General anaesthetics are to be avoided.

ENCEPHALITIS

This is inflammation of the brain most commonly complicating viral infections, such as herpes, influenza, mumps and measles. It is a serious condition characterized by fever, headache, vomiting, confusion, convulsions, coma and, occasionally, death. Permanent brain damage of varying degree occurs in a significant number of patients and epilepsy may result.

In most cases there is no specific treatment although antiviral agents are sometimes used.

Treatment is supportive and symptomatic.

Dental significance

There is no dental significance.

ENDOCARDITIS

For endocarditis, *see under* Heart disease, infective – Infective endocarditis.

ENTERIC FEVER

For enteric fever, *see* Typhoid.

EPIDEMIC MYALGIA

For epidemic myalgia, *see* Bornholm's disease.

EPIGLOTITIS

This uncommon, but life-threatening, condition of children is of acute onset. It starts with a sore throat and signs of an upper respiratory infection which rapidly progress to airway obstruction. Both inspiration and expiration are noisy and laboured and the child has to sit up to breathe. In over 90% of cases, the causative organism is *Haemophilus influenzae* type B.

Treatment is urgent hospital admission, intubation under a general anaesthetic and intravenous antibiotics, usually *chloramphenicol.* The administration of oxygen can be an important interim measure.

Dental significance

There is no dental significance, but dentists should be aware of the condition and its severity.

EPILEPSY

This is a recurrent disturbance of electrical activity of the brain resulting in symptoms which include impairment of consciousness, convulsive moments, sensory abnormalities and psychic disturbances. Epilepsy may follow brain damage from any cause, trauma, cerebrovascular accidents, infection, ischaemia, anoxia or malignancy, but most commonly there is no obvious cause.

An international classification of epilepsy was agreed by a commission of the International League against Epilepsy in 1969 and adopted subsequently by the World Health Organisation. This classification divides the clinical presentations of epilepsy into:

1. Generalized (which includes grand mal, petit mal and the myoclonic epilepsies).
2. Partial (which included temporal lobe and focal seizures).
3. Miscellaneous (which includes photosensitive epilepsy).

General epilepsy

Grand mal

Typically there is an initial aura, followed by the tonic stage with loss of consciousness, a brief cessation of respiration and cyanosis. After this the clonic stage occurs with convulsive movements affecting the trunk, limbs, jaw, and tongue; in this stage the patient may froth at the mouth, bite the tongue and be incontinent. Coma follows, lasting minutes to hours. Recovery is often accompanied by headache and occasionally post-epileptic automatism.

Petit mal

These attacks consist of brief periods of loss of consciousness when the patient stops what he is doing or saying for a few seconds and then carries on.

Partial epilepsy

This results from focal electrical discharges, the clinical manifestations depending on the site involved. They may be so minor as to pass unnoticed. Temporal lobe epilepsy results from electrical discharge in the temporal lobe resulting in organized movements, sensations or emotions.

In recent years, *carbamazepine* (Tegretol$_{GB,US}$) and *sodium valproate* (Epilim$_{GB}$, Depakene$_{US}$), have taken over as first-line drugs from the more conventional *phenytoin* and *phenobarbitone*. *Carbamazepine* is the drug of choice for partial seizures and tonic–clonic seizures with partial onset, and is relatively free of side-effects. *Phenytoin* is still widely used and is very effective in treatment of tonic–clonic seizures. However, it has disadvantages, especially in the younger age groups, causing hirsutism, coarsening of the facies, gum hypertrophy and acne. *Phenobarbitone* (Luminal$_{GB}$) is effective and may be valuable where other drugs have failed to control epilepsy. However, it should not be a drug of first choice as it causes sedation and, in the elderly, confusion and depression.

Status epilepticus

Seizures occasionally follow one after the other without remission. When these are tonic–clonic (grand mal) seizures, the patient is at great risk of brain damage or death through cardiorespiratory failure, unless the attacks are stopped.

Although not drugs of choice for ordinary epileptic attacks, intravenous *diazepam* (Valium$_{GB,US}$), *lorazepam* (Ativan$_{GB,US}$) or *clonazepam* (Rivotril$_{GB}$, Clonopin$_{US}$) are extremely effective in status epilepticus, given as a bolus injection. If *diazepam* is given, 10 mg in 2 ml intravenously, given over 2–5 minutes, is recommended. Larger doses may cause respiratory depression. If the attack is not stopped, an infusion of *diazepam* 200 mg in 1 litre of saline may be given, the infusion rate being adjusted to control the fits.

Dental significance

There are no contraindications to routine dentisty in epileptics. For those who suffer from grand mal, loose-fitting partial dentures are inadvisable. Anaesthetic agents may be administered to epileptics in the dental surgery.

Fibrous hyperplasia of the gingivae occurs in 50% of patients treated with *phenytoin* (Epanutin$_{GB}$, Dilantin$_{US}$). It seems to be unrelated to dosage but is commoner in the young. The underlying mechanism is not understood but meticulous plaque control helps to reduce the problem. Delayed eruption and permanent teeth of diminished size have been reported in epileptics treated with this drug since a young age.

If a dentist is called to a patient having an attack of 'grand mal' epilepsy, he should seek assistance to hold the patient on his side on the floor. Until the clonic stage has passed, the patient should be gently refrained from hurting himself. Props to prevent tongue biting are best avoided. He should then be kept warm and allowed to rest until full consciousness has returned.

Epileptics will know about their condition and are embarrassed by over-zealous and unnecessary after-care. Provided cyanosis was not prolonged and the patient is fully recovered and uninjured, he or she may be allowed to leave, but should be accompanied home.

EPILOIA

For epiloia, *see* Tuberous sclerosis.

ERYSIPELAS

This is a skin infection caused by a group A streptococcus. It usually involves the face and head but may occur elsewhere beginning as an abrupt fever. A zone of redness and oedema occurs commonly on the bridge of the nose or around wounds, trauma sites or an area of dermatitis. The facial lesion may spread to involve most of the face. Treatment is with *penicillin*.

Dental significance

The condition is not of dental origin but dentists should recognize it as patients may consult them, thinking it is.

ERYTHEMA MULTIFORME

This condition, mostly seen in young adults, is a reaction pattern in the skin and mucous membrane causing erythematous lesions which may be oedematous or bullous, darkening with age to give the characteristic target lesions. It has been associated with infections such as herpes simplex, with vaccination, drugs and malignancy, but in one-third of cases the cause is not known. The condition may present as a minor disease with few lesions or as a major life-threatening disease (*see* Stevens–Johnson syndrome).

Dental significance

The condition may present to the dentist as haemorrhagic bullae round the lips and in the mouth which quickly break down to ulcers. Among the drugs used in dentistry, which are thought to be responsible factors are: *barbiturates, carbamazepine* (Tegretol$_{GB, US}$), *penicillin* and *sulphonamides* (Bactrim$_{GB, US}$ and Septrin$_{GB}$). The condition is self-limiting, but topical steroids in the form of *hydrocortisone* pellets (Corlan$_{GB}$) four times daily after meals, or *triamcinolone* (Adcortyl$_{GB}$, Kenalog$_{US}$) in orobase, will be helpful.

ERYTHEMA NODOSUM

This is considered to be a hypersensitivity vasculitis resulting in painful red nodules one or more centimetres in diameter. Most commonly these occur on the legs but are also seen on the arms. The condition is associated with infections such as tuberculosis, leprosy and streptococcal infections; with sarcoid, inflammatory bowel disease and with such drugs as *sulphonamides*. It is self-limiting. Treatment involves management of the underlying cause and treatment of symptoms.

Dental significance

There is no dental significance.

FALLOT'S TETRALOGY

For Fallot's tetralogy, *see under* Heart disease, congenital.

FAMILIAL HYPERCHOLESTEROLAEMIA

For familial hypercholesterolaemia, *see* Hyperlipidaemias.

FAMILIAL PERIODIC PARALYSIS

This condition is characterized by recurrent attacks of flaccid weakness usually associated with hypokalaemia but occasionally hyperkalaemia. It is described in families with an autosomal dominant pattern of inheritance. Sporadic cases are seen. Diagnosis is based on a typical history and abnormal potassium levels in the serum.

Treatment of hypokalaemia is with oral potassium chloride 5–10 g. Recovery is usual in half an hour but may take hours. Hyperkalaemic paralysis requires an infusion of glucose and insulin. As a preventative treatment, *acetazolamide* ($\text{Diamox}_{\text{GB, US}}$) has been found effective in both hyper- and hypokalaemic paralysis. (*See* Hypokalaemic periodic paralysis.)

Dental significance

There is no dental significance.

FARMER'S LUNG

For farmer's lung, *see* Pneumoconioses.

FIBROCYSTIC DISEASE

For fibrocystic disease, *see* Cystic fibrosis.

FOOT AND MOUTH DISEASE

This virus disease is highly infectious among cattle, sheep and pigs, but seldom contracted by humans. The incubation period is 2–5 days and painful vesicles occur in the mouth and spread to other parts of the body, notably palms of hands and soles of feet. Diagnosis can be confirmed by laboratory examination of fluid from the vesicles.

Dental significance

Although painful, the disease is not dangerous and clears up in 1–2 weeks. Secondary infection of oral lesions can be prevented by use of *erythromycin* mouthwash (5 ml of Erythroped$_{GB}$ or Ilosone$_{GB,US}$ 25 mg to 1 ml) in children and *tetracycline* and *amphotericin* mouthwash (5 ml Mysteclin$_{GB,US}$) in adults.

FRIEDREICH'S ATAXIA

This heredofamilial disorder presents in the first or second decade with unsteadiness, clumsiness, dysarthria, then weakness and ataxia. Additional features on examination include nystagmus, absent knee and ankle jerks, extensor plantar reflexes, optic atrophy, pes cavus, scoliosis and cardiac arrhythmias.

There is no treatment.

Dental significance

Nothing specifically associated with the disorder but assistance with oral hygiene may be required.

GALLBLADDER DISEASE

For gallbladder disease, *see* Biliary disease.

GALLSTONES

For gallstones, *see under* Biliary disease.

GASTRIC ULCER

For gastric ulcer, *see* Peptic ulceration.

GASTRITIS

Acute gastritis

This is a diffuse inflammation of the gastric mucosa resulting from various factors: alcohol, aspirin and anti-inflammatory drugs. In most cases the cause is poorly understood. The symptoms are epigastric discomfort, nausea and loss of appetite.

Treatment is similar to that for peptic ulceration.

Atrophic gastritis

This is a chronic inflammation of the stomach resulting in gastric mucosal atrophy and achlorhydria, leading to pernicious anaemia.

Dental significance

With atrophy of the gastric mucosa, secretion of intrinsic factor (of Castle) is diminished and this results in failure to absorb vitamin B_{12}. Together with a megaloblastic anaemia the patient may suffer from a painful atrophic glossitis and recurrent oral ulceration.

GASTROENTERITIS

This is a clinical syndrome of diarrhoea and vomiting associated with gastrointestinal infection, either viral or bacterial. Most attacks last no more than a few days and are self-limiting. They commonly result from ingestion of contaminated water or food where hygiene is poor. Symptomatic treatment is usually all that is required. In general, antibiotics do not affect the course of the disease and may delay clearance of the organism from the gut. Some studies have suggested that prophylactic use of broad-spectrum antibiotics such as *sulphatriad* (a compound *sulphonamide*) may reduce attack rate. The best preventative measures are largely common sense: when in areas of poor hygiene, boil drinking water, avoid salad, peel fruit, don't buy it precut and take great care with personal hygiene.

Dental significance

A furred tongue, with accompanying dry mouth, is a common feature.

GAUCHER'S DISEASE

This is a familial disorder resulting in an abnormal accumulation of glycocerebrocides in the reticuloendothelial cells. Three syndromes are recognized:

1. A chronic adult form with hyperplenism, bone lesions, pinguecu-lae and skin pigmentation – this is the most common form.
2. An acute neuropathic form seen in infancy, and usually fatal.
3. A juvenile form combining features of the chronic form with progressive neurological dysfunctions.

There is no specific treatment.

Dental significance

Radiotranslucent areas have been reported in the mandible. Nasal and gingival bleeding may occur, with excessive haemorrhage following dental extractions.

GERMAN MEASLES

For German measles, *see* Rubella.

GIANT CELL ARTERITIS

This condition results from a granulomatous arteritis and is confined to the elderly. Severe headache and scalp tenderness are the cardinal features, although symptoms may be very similar to those of polymyalgia rheumatica. Discomfort in the temporalis and masseter muscles together with stiffness of the jaw is not uncommon. Occasionally, fever and malaise are the only features. It is usual for the erythrocyte sedimentation rate (ESR) to be raised. The all-important complication is the rapid development of blindness and, as soon as the diagnosis is made, urgent treatment with systemic steroids is mandatory. Diagnosis is confirmed by temporal artery biopsy. Dosage of steroids can be sometimes cut down by the use of *azathioprine* (Imuran$_{GB,US}$) in a dosage of 100 mg or 150 mg daily.

Dental significance

As in polymyalgia rheumatica, jaw-ache and tenderness of masseter and temporal muscles may be a prominent complaint, and it is not uncommon for those with these problems to consult their dentist. If no dental cause can be found and the patient's age and symptoms point to giant cell arteritis being a possible diagnosis, they should be referred to their doctor for confirmation and treatment before eye damage occurs. Dentists should enquire if corticosteroids have been taken in the last 3 months and act accordingly (*see* Adrenal insufficiency).

GIANT URTICARIA

For giant urticaria, *see* Angio-oedema.

GIARDIASIS

This is a gastrointestinal infection caused by the protozoan *Giardia lamblia*. It occurs world wide, not just in the tropics but in any area of poor hygiene. Many holidaymakers in Leningrad seem to contract the infection. It may present as an acute illness with diarrhoea, nausea, abdominal pain and vomiting, or as a chronic diarrhoeal illness.

Diagnosis depends on demonstrating cysts in the stool or the protozoa in jejunal juice.

Treatment

The drug of choice is *metronidazole* (Flagyl$_{GB,US}$) 400 mg 8-hourly for 7 days.

Dental significance

There is no dental significance.

GILBERT'S SYNDROME

The importance of this condition is in differentiating it from other causes of jaundice because it is entirely benign and of no clinical significance once correctly diagnosed. The important features are mild jaundice and a modest rise in unconjugated bilirubin in the blood. The condition is seen in between 3% and 7% of the general population and is more common in men. It is due to a congenital defect in hepatic bile clearance from the circulation. The cause is not known.

Dental significance

There is no dental significance.

GLANDULAR FEVER

For glandular fever, *see* Infectious mononucleosis.

GLAUCOMA

Glaucoma is a rise in intraocular pressure sufficient to cause degeneration of the optic disc and visual field defects. It is a leading cause of acquired blindness estimated to occur in 2% of adults over 40.

The condition may be primary (open-angle), secondary or congenital. Primary glaucoma is a slowly progressive bilateral disease of insidious onset and, if undetected and untreated, leads to progressive loss of visual field and blindness. Treatment is usually medical and prognosis good. Congenital glaucoma is due to anterior segment anomalies. Symptoms are dramatic with the onset of sudden severe pain, nausea and vomiting with blurring of vision. Attacks may be precipitated by mydriatics such as *atropine*. Such drugs should not be used if glaucoma is suspected.

Treatment is with *pilocarpine* and *timolol* eye drops. Iridectomy is indicated when medical treatment fails.

Dental significance

Even today many cases of glaucoma are undetected until too late and dentists should advise patients at risk to have their eyes examined. Risk factors include family history, increasing age, myopia, diabetes and coronary disease.

A dentist should always enquire if a patient suffers from glaucoma before giving *atropine* in any form.

GLOMERULONEPHRITIS

For glomerulonephritis, *see under* Renal disease.

GLOSSOPHARYNGEAL NEURALGIA

This is a rare form of neuralgia comparable to trigeminal neuralgia in the characteristics of the pain. It most commonly affects the elderly and may be felt deep in the ear or in the throat. Treatment with *carbamazepine* (Tegretol$_{GB,US}$) may be effective.

Dental significance

With the symptoms related to the throat and ear, the condition is less likely to be confused with a dental pathology.

GONORRHOEA

This is a venereal disease due to the gonococcus *Neisseria gonorrhoeae*. It it usually acquired by coitus with an infected person. The incubation period of 3–10 days is followed by dysuria, a purulent urethral discharge, and tender groin glands. In men the prostate and seminal vesicles may be involved and in women Bartholin's gland, the uterus and fallopian tubes may become infected leading to permanent sterility. Septic arthritis may complicate the infection. Infection does not convey immunity.

Treatment is with *procaine penicillin* with *probenecid* (Benemid$_{GB,US}$). However, resistant strains of the gonococcus are now common, accounting for the increased failure rate of conventional treatment.

Dental significance

Gonorrhoeal stomatitis or tonsillitis can result from direct infection through oral sex with an infected partner, by autotransfer from a patient's genital infection, or as part of a disseminated gonococcal infection. Painful inflammation and oedema of the mucous membrane is usual, ulceration less common. Arthritis of the temporomandibular joint is a rare complication.

Diagnosis is not possible from a direct smear and culture from a swab of exudate is necessary.

Treatment is with *procaine penicillin* 600 mg i.m. daily and *probenecid* (Benemid$_{GB, US}$) 250 mg twice daily for 1 week.

GOUT

This clinical syndrome results from a rise in the serum uric acid level. The cause of the rise may be an excessive synthesis as is postulated in primary or genetic gout, and as is seen in conditions of excessive tissue turnover, lymphomata and leukaemia. The alternative cause is reduced renal clearance most commonly seen in renal failure, and as a complication of the use of certain drugs, e.g. thiazide diuretics.

The main clinical feature is acute arthritis most commonly affecting the first metatarsophalangeal joints. Crystal deposits are seen in the skin as gouty tophi. The condition is complicated by renal crystal deposits leading to infection and renal damage.

Treatment of the acute attacks is with *indomethacin* (Indocid$_{GB}$, Indocin$_{US}$). Preventative treatment involves avoidance of drugs known to precipitate gout and the use of the xanthine oxidase inhibitor *allopurinol* (Zyloric$_{GB}$, Lopurin$_{US}$, Zyloprim$_{US}$).

Dental significance

The arthritis of gout may involve the temporomandibular joint, and if so a soft bite block will make the patient more comfortable.

GRAVE'S DISEASE

For Grave's disease, *see* Thyroid disease.

GUILLAIN–BARRÉ SYNDROME

This syndrome is an acute neuropathy, predominantly motor, of uncertain aetiology. Most probably there is a cell-mediated immune response provoked by certain viral infections, and directed at normal peripheral myelin. There is frequently a history of an infective illness, viral in nature, in the preceding few weeks. Progressive weakness occurs over 2–3 weeks commonly affecting the lower limbs first, but the arms and cranial nerves are frequently affected and involvement of muscles of respiration may necessitate ventilation.

Recovery is usual, but 20% of patients are left with residual disability. The cerebrospinal fluid protein is usually raised although the cell count is normal.

There is no specific treatment. Management consists of careful nursing, physiotherapy and a continuous awareness of the possible need of artificial ventilation.

Dental significance

Weakness in muscles of mastication, with difficulty in chewing, has been reported.

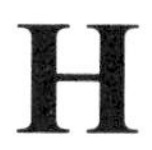

HAEMOCHROMATOSIS

For haemochromatosis, *see under* Liver disease – Cirrhosis.

HAEMOPHILIA, CHRISTMAS DISEASE AND VON WILLEBRAND'S DISEASE

These inherited blood coagulation disorders are caused by a partial or complete deficiency of one or several factors which are essential for normal haemostasis and whose absence results in persistent haemorrhage. Factor VIII is missing in haemophilia, factor IX in Christmas disease and factor VIII, together with von Willebrand's factor, in von Willebrand's disease. Of the three, haemophilia is most common with an incidence of 5 in every 100 000 individuals. The condition is inherited as an X-linked recessive trait, transmitted by females, some of whom may bleed excessively, and evident in males.

While the precise diagnosis is made by specific plasma assay of the individual factors, the clinical history is of great importance. Severe haemophiliacs have a plasma level of factor VIII of 0–1% (normal range, 45–200%) and suffer haemorrhages sometimes for little or no apparent reason. In less severe haemophilia with factor VIII levels of 2–5%, joint haemorrhages and continued bleeding occur, usually after trauma, while in 'mild' haemophilia with factor VIII levels of 5–30% excessive bleeding will only be apparent with operations or major trauma but may then be troublesome.

Dental significance

At the present time in the UK, it is to be expected that all sufferers will be under the care and guidance of a haemophilia centre and dental treatment should only be undertaken after consulting medical staff at the centre.

In patients with mild to moderate haemophilia, conservative treatment can usually be carried out without supplements of the missing factor or antifibrinolytic agent providing the following points are observed: nerve block anaesthesia must be avoided but infiltration injections of local anaesthetic may be permissible and this can be supplemented when required by sedation or the use of oral analgesics. Haematomata in the floor of the mouth can result from the use of saliva ejectors and bite wing X-ray holders and the floor of the mouth should be protected with gauze when using these. Scaling and cavity preparation should be undertaken with extra care to avoid laceration of the gingiva and, in root treatment, the dentist must take care not to ream through the apex.

Before contemplating extractions or other oral surgery, assessment of the patient's factor VIII level must be undertaken and the presence of factor VIII antibody excluded. The HIV antibody and hepatitis B antigen status should also be determined. Then with the participation of the haemophilia centre, steps are taken to increase the factor level to that sufficient to produce and maintain adequate haemostasis. Usually this means admission to hospital and the giving of the missing factor together with the antifibrinolytic agent *tranexamic acid* preoperatively and, in the majority of cases, post-operative *tranexamic acid* only for a period of 10 days by mouth. In some cases where the factor VIII:C level is not too low and depending on the surgery involved, the factor VIII level can be elevated by an intravenous injection of *1-desamino-8-D-arginine vasopressin* (desmopressin, DDAVP) together with *tranexamic acid* and this form of therapy may make unnecessary the exposure of the patient to blood products. The prescription of analgesics containing *aspirin* is contraindicated before or after surgery as the use of even a small dose of aspirin may interfere with platelet function for a considerable time and so increase the chances of postoperative bleeding or facial bruising. The same comment would apply to non-steroidal anti-inflammatory drugs.

As a result of screening of blood donors and the heat treatment of factor concentrates, the risk of haemophiliacs becoming HIV positive or carriers of hepatitis is now very small. However, a number have been infected in the past with these conditions and, if so, their dental treatment should be conducted with precautions as described under AIDS and hepatitis (*see* Liver disease).

HAND, FOOT AND MOUTH DISEASE

The disease is caused by infection with the Coxsackie A virus, has an incubation period of 3–6 days, and is seen mainly in young children. Painful ulcers occur in the mouth and vesicles on the palmar surface of the hands and plantar surface of the feet. There is usually mild pyrexia and malaise. The condition resolves in about 10 days. There is no treatment.

Dental significance

Antiseptic lozenges containing a local anaesthetic will ease the patient's discomfort and prevent secondary infection. It is likely that the virus is present in exudate from the ulcers so care should be taken in sterilizing instruments and the rinse-out glass.

HANSEN'S DISEASE

For Hansen's disease, *see* Leprosy.

HASHIMOTO'S DISEASE

For Hashimoto's disease, *see under* Thyroid disease.

HEART DISEASE, CONGENITAL

Atrial septal defect

An atrial septal defect (ASD) of the ostium secundum type is a common developmental cardiac abnormality resulting in a left-to-right heart shunt. It often gives rise to no symptoms until adult life when dyspnoea and palpitations due to extrasystoles or atrial fibrillation occur. The important complication is pulmonary hypertension which may lead to shunt reversal and cyanosis. The ostium primum ASD is much rarer and associated with mitral incompetence and left axis deviation on the ECG.

Treatment is surgical for moderate to large shunts and contraindicated with severe pulmonary hypertension.

Dental significance

Patients with open or repaired atrial defects should receive antibiotic cover for all procedures likely to cause a bacteraemia (*see* Heart disease, infective – Infective endocarditis). With those having small or repaired defects it is safe to give a general anaesthetic in the surgery, but reduced exercise tolerance requires the administration of anaesthetics in hospital.

Fallot's tetralogy

The anatomical features of this condition are pulmonary stenosis, a high ventricular septal defect, an overriding aorta and right ventricular hypertrophy. It is the commonest form of congenital cyanotic heart disease. Complete surgical repair is the treatment of choice.

Dental significance

Antibiotic cover is mandatory for all dental procedures likely to cause a bacteraemia (*see under* Heart disease, infective – Infective endocarditis). General anaesthetics should only be administered in hospital.

Patent ductus arteriosus

This is a developmental abnormality where a fetal channel between the aorta and main pulmonary artery persists. It is commonly asymptomatic but if large may lead to dyspnoea and palpitations. Examination reveals a loud continuous murmur (Gibson or machinery murmur). Pulmonary hypertension and infective endocarditis are complications of the untreated condition. Treatment is surgical and curative if performed before complications occur.

Dental significance

Antibiotic cover for procedures likely to cause a bacteraemia is probably wise, but for patients in whom the defect has been treated, the risk is small (*see under* Heart disease, infective – Infective endocarditis). A small asymptomatic patent ductus, or one which has been successfully closed, does not mitigate against general anaesthetics in the surgery.

Ventricular septal defect

This defect (VSD) may involve the membranous or muscular part of the septum. Small defects produce no disability and are compatible with a normal life, while larger ones lead to heart failure, the degree of shunt depending on the size of the defect. Auscultation reveals a loud pansystolic murmur. The major complications are pulmonary hypertension and infective endocarditis. Pyogenic infections and dental procedures should be covered by antibiotics. Patients with small shunts can lead normal lives while surgery is the treatment of choice for larger defects.

Dental significance

All dental procedures likely to cause a bacteraemia should receive antibiotic cover (*see under* Heart disease, infective – Infective endocarditis). General anaesthetics should be administered in hospital.

Coarctation of the aorta

Coarctation results from a developmental abnormality of the aortic arch. Diagnostic features are high arterial pressures in the upper limbs with lower pressure and delayed pulses in the lower limbs. The important associations are arterial hypertension resulting in cerebral arterial lesions and aortic valve disease. Treatment is surgical correction, without which the average age of death is 35 years.

Dental significance

Antibiotic cover should be given for all procedures likely to cause a bacteraemia (*see under* Heart disease, infective – Infective endocarditis). General anaesthetics should be avoided and, if essential, administered in hospital.

HEART DISEASE, DYSRHYTHMIAS

Atrial fibrillation

This results from multiple ectopic foci discharging rapidly, producing very rapid atrial rates of 400/minute or more. The ventricles are unable to respond to this rate and respond at a variable rate between 60 and 200 due to variable electrical block. Most commonly it results from ischaemic heart disease but may be due to thyrotoxicosis, pneumonia or valvular heart disease.

Ventricular rate is controlled with *digoxin*. Systemic embolization is the main hazard. Heart failure may complicate uncontrolled fibrillation.

Dental significance

Aspirating syringes and local anaesthetics without adrenaline should be used in these patients. Antibiotic cover will not be required unless there is a history of rheumatic or congenital heart disease, in which case it should be given for 'at-risk' procedures as described in Heart disease, infective – Infective endocarditis. Unless the condition is fully controlled, anaesthetics should only be administered in hospital.

Paroxysmal atrial tachycardia

Commonly atrial or supraventricular, these paroxysms, arising from a single ectopic focus, come on suddenly and usually result in a pulse rate between 150 and 220/minute. The duration is from minutes to days. Although sometimes associated with underlying heart disease, commonly the heart is normal. They occur at any age and may be associated with anomalous atrioventricular conduction as in the

Wolff–Parkinson–White (WPW) syndrome, where premature ventricular excitation occurs due to conduction via an anomalous pathway to the ventricles. The ECG may be normal or show the characteristic short P–R interval. In the absence of underlying heart disease, the prognosis is excellent. Treatment consists of reassurance. Usually attacks cease spontaneously, but carotid sinus massage is sometimes effective in arresting the attack. When prolonged antidysrhythmic agents such as *verapamil* (Cordilox$_{GB}$) are indicated.

Dental significance

There are no contraindications to routine dental treatment. General anaesthetics may be administered to patients who suffer from this condition provided there is no underlying heart disease and the pulse is normal at the time. Commensurate treatment with *verapamil* may potentiate the hypotensive effect of anaesthetic agents.

Heart block

The term 'heart block' describes a situation where the conduction of electrical excitation from the atria is delayed at the junctional tissues (the AV node and the bundle of His). On the ECG, the P–R interval is the time taken for the impulse to travel from the atria across the junctional tissue and down the ventricular bundles. In its mildest form (first-degree heart block), the P–R interval is abnormally prolonged (greater than 0.2 second). As conduction deteriorates, periodic impulses fail to cross to the ventricles and no ventricular beat occurs (second-degree block). In its most extreme form (third-degree block, complete heart block or AV dissociation), no impulses pass from atria to ventricles and both beat independently of one another.

The commonest cause of heart block is ischaemic heart disease although it may result from viral infection, infiltrative disease such as amyloid, collagen disorders, cardiomyopathies and, occasionally, it may be congenital. The prognosis of first- and second-degree heart block is favourable although this clearly depends on the underlying cause. The outcome in complete heart block is unpredictable and, because of the high risk of cardiac standstill or ventricular fibrillation leading to Stokes–Adams attacks, any of which may be fatal, cardiac pacing is usually recommended. In the presence of Stokes–Adams attacks pacing is a matter of urgency, a temporary pacemaker being inserted until a permanent pacemaker can be implanted.

Cardiac pacemakers

Transvenous endocardial pacing is the method used for temporary pacing and the transvenous route is favoured for permanent pacing also. The two principal modes of pacing are fixed rate, when pacing is preset and occurs independently of intrinsic heart rate, and demand pacing when the pacemaker fires only when the ventricular rate falls below a predetermined level. The latter method is safer and the preferred method.

Dental significance

Research has shown that diathermy and the magnetostrictive types of ultrasonic scalers can affect the function of pacemakers if in close proximity, and their use is therefore inadvisable. Although the risk is not high, antibiotic cover should be given to patients with pacemakers for procedures likely to cause a bacteraemia (*see under* Heart disease, infective – Infective endocarditis).

General anaesthetics should be administered in hospital.

Stokes–Adams attack

This is a sudden loss of consciousness due to transient circulatory arrest resulting from ventricular asystole or tachycardia. It is almost invariably associated with underlying ischaemic heart disease particularly when complete heart block is present. Attacks may be infrequent or multiple in rapid succession. When associated with complete heart block, permanent cardiac pacing is indicated.

Dental significance

General anaesthetics are to be avoided, but if essential administered in hospital.

HEART DISEASE, INFECTIVE

Infective endocarditis

This was formerly known as subacute bacterial endocarditis (SBE). Infective endocarditis may be caused by bacteria or fungal infection and may present acutely or subacutely.

Acute infective endocarditis usually results from infection by pyogenic bacteria such as *Staphylococcus aureus* or *Streptococcus pneumoniae*. The disease may occur in the absence of pre-existing heart disease and progress rapidly with tissue destruction and abscess formation to cardiac failure. The mortality rate is high, death occurs early in the course of the disease and is often not influenced by medical or surgical intervention.

Subacute infective endocarditis, by contrast, usually presents with chronic ill health over weeks or months, and diagnosis is frequently missed on account of the wide variety of ways in which it may present. The commonest organism is *Streptococcus viridans* and there is usually underlying cardiac pathology. Prognosis is better than for acute endocarditis, provided the diagnosis is made and adequate treatment given.

Specific symptoms are a result of emboli from valve cusp vegetations lodging in cerebral and peripheral vessels, and from valvular destruction leading to heart failure. Important clinical features are: fever, anaemia, splinter haemorrhage, haematuria, splenomegaly and changing heart murmurs. A high ESR and a normochromic anaemia support the diagnosis, which is confirmed by blood cultures.

Antibiotic therapy depends on the organism and its sensitivity. Bactericidal antibodies must be used. Streptococcal pneumonia requires treatment with high dose *benzylpenicillin* 9.0–12 g i.v. per day alone or with *gentamicin*. *Streptococcus viridans* is usually highly sensitive to *penicillin*. Treatment is started with *benzylpenicillin* 7 g i.v. per day together with *gentamicin* 40 mg twice daily for 2 weeks. Thereafter, *benzylpenicillin* is continued alone intravenously for a further 2 weeks.

Dental significance

Extractions and some other dental procedures would appear to be important predisposing factors in this condition. Having said that, endocarditis following dental treatment is rare, only occurring in a small proportion of 'at-risk' patients after dental treatment. However, in view of the mortality of the disease, it is the duty of dentists to take reasonable measures towards its prevention.

Although it is possible for almost any dental procedure to evoke a bacteraemia, for practical purposes those for which antibiotic cover should be given to patients at risk are: tooth extraction and oral surgery involving the gingiva, scaling and endodontic treatment where there is a danger of forcing infected debris through the apex. Patients at risk fall into the following groups:

1. Patients with congenital heart disease, including septal defects, bicuspid aortic valves and patent ductus arteriosus.
2. Patients with rheumatic fever or postrheumatic valvular heart disease.
3. Patients with prosthetic heart valves.

4. Patients who have previously suffered fro
   carditis.

Patients in the last two categories should be
risk cases and are best referred to hospital for
they are not allergic to *penicillin* and have not
the last month, patients in categories (1) and (2
local anaesthetic should be given *amoxycillin*
mouth 1 hour before treatment. The dose should
under 10 and 750 mg if under 5 years of age. Those allergi
penicillin, or those who have received *penicillin* during the last month should be given *erythromycin* (Erythrocin$_{GB, US}$, Ilosone$_{GB, US}$) 1.5 g by mouth 1–2 hours before and a second dose of 0.5 g 6 hours later. Half the dose should be given to children under 10 and a quarter of the dose to those under 5 years of age. Patients who require treatment under a general anaesthetic, but are not allergic to *penicillin* or have not received it during the last month should be given *amoxycillin* (Amoxil injection$_{GB, US}$) 1.0 g i.m. 1 hour before and 0.5 g by mouth 6 hours afterwards. Those requiring a general anaesthetic, who are allergic to *penicillin* or have received it in the last month are best referred to hospital for treatment, which will have to be carried out under cover of intravenous *vancomycin* and *gentamicin*.

Any effort to reduce oral infection such as pre-extraction mouthwashes of *chlorhexidine* (Corsodyl$_{GB}$, Peridex$_{US}$) is worth instituting, and patients at risk should be advised to consult their doctors if they feel unwell in the subsequent 2 or 3 months.

Those who have undergone angioplasty or by-pass operations are not considered to be at risk.

HEART DISEASE, ISCHAEMIC

Angina pectoris

This term describes the symptom of myocardial ischaemia. It results when the heart muscle becomes critically short of oxygen, usually due to coronary artery atheroma. It may be aggravated by anaemia and anoxia. It is usually brought on by exercise but may occur unrelated to activity (unstable angina).

The main lines of treatment are:

1. Vasodilator drugs such as short- and long-acting nitrates, e.g. *glyceryl trinitrate* and *isosorbide dinitrate*.
2. β-Adrenoceptor blocking drugs which reduce cardiac work such as *propranolol* (Inderal$_{GB, US}$) and *atenolol* (Tenormin$_{GB, US}$).
3. Calcium channel blockers such as *nifedipine* (Adalat$_{GB, US}$) or *diltiazem* (Tildiem$_{GB}$, Cardizem$_{US}$).

dial infarction

e than quarter of a million heart attacks occur each year in the K and 40% of patients die during the 4 weeks following their heart attack; 25% of these deaths are instantaneous. The cause of death is usually ventricular fibrillation. The pain from myocardial infarction is similar to anginal pain but very much more severe and persistent. However, very occasionally myocardial infarction is painless.

Dental significance

Patients with a history of angina pectoris or myocardial infarction may be treated in a general dental practice with a few precautions. But if a patient has suffered a myocardial infarction, surgical procedures should be delayed for 3 months if possible.

General anaesthetics should be avoided, and painful conservative work and surgery carried out with local anaesthesia. A local anaesthetic solution without a vasoconstrictor should be employed, and intravenous injection avoided by use of an aspirating syringe. Haemostatic string or pack containing *adrenaline* should not be used. Care to avoid anxiety and stress is important, and oral or intravenous sedatives should be used where necessary.

Patients who use *nitrates* to ease their symptoms should bring the drugs into the surgery with them.

If on anticoagulant therapy (*warfarin* or other anticoagulants), extractions or other surgery must only be undertaken after consultation with the patient's doctor or specialist. It the patient's life is not put at risk thereby, the anticoagulant treatment must be discontinued or reduced prior to surgery and a clotting time or prothrombin estimation checked to make sure that these figures are within normal limits.

Cases of gingival hyperplasia, similar to that seen with *phenytoin*, have been reported in patients treated with *nifedipine* (Adalat$_{\text{GB, US}}$).

Cardiac arrest

This is most commonly due to myocardial infarction but may occasionally complicate hypoxia due to an anaesthetic accident. Asystole may occur but more commonly the arrest results from ventricular fibrillation. Although the diagnosis is usually obvious, cardiac arrest is recognized by the following features: collapse, loss of consciousness, pallor, loss of pulses and apnoea.

Management

Speed is essential; irreversible brain damage results within 3–5 minutes of arrest. The following manoeuvres should be carried out:

1. Lay the patient flat on the floor, face upwards.
2. Clear airway, remove dentures, loosen collar, insert airway if available, send assistant to call for ambulance.
3. Apply sharp blow with the hand to the lower sternum – in the case of a dysrhythmia this may restart the heart.
4. Commence external cardiac massage and mouth-to-mouth respiration. Place flat of right hand over lower half of sternum, place left hand on top of right hand, kneel beside patient, deliver five forcible thrusts to the chest at approximately 1-second intervals. Ventilate by closing the patient's nostrils with finger and thumb, inhaling deeply, and exhaling through patient's mouth.

This sequence of events should be repeated until assistance comes. Ventilation is more effective using an airway and Ambu bag and preferably oxygen.

Prosthetic heart valves

The three types of prosthetic heart valves, in use today, are the Starr–Edwards (a ball and cage), the Björk–Shiley (a low profile tilting disc) and the porcine xenograft (a mounted pig's aortic valve). The former two require lifelong anticoagulation, but for the porcine xenograft, which is becoming increasingly popular, anticoagulants are usually not required, provided it is mounted in either the mitral or aortic position and in a patient with sinus rhythm.

Dental significance

All dental procedures likely to cause a bacteraemia should be undertaken with antibiotic cover (*see under* Heart disease, infective – Infective endocarditis) and, if the patient is receiving anticoagulants (*warfarin* or other anticoagulants), an estimation of the patient's clotting time should be undertaken before surgery, and if the clotting time (Lee White) exceeds 20 minutes the patient referred to hospital.

It should be appreciated that short-acting barbiturates induce the liver microsomal enzymes which degrade *warfarin* and, therefore, effective anticoagulation may be lost. In consequence, dental treatment under barbiturate sedation is best avoided.

HEMIBALLISM (HEMICHOREA)

Hemiballism describes a wild flinging movement of one arm or leg, being irregular in timing and force. Although it may be seen in association with Sydenham's chorea in the young, it most commonly occurs in elderly hypertensive diabetic patients as a consequence of a vascular lesion in the subthalamic nucleus on the contralateral side. Rarely, a tumour at the same site may cause hemiballism. When associated with a stroke, the hemiballism usually remits spontaneously over 3–6 months.

Treatment is with *phenothiazine* or stereotactic surgery.

Dental significance

It goes without saying that dental treatment has to be tailored to the severity of the patient's condition, always appreciating that the uncontrolled movements are likely to abate with the passage of time. The association with diabetes and vascular disease must not be forgotten.

HEMIFACIAL SPASM

This condition, mainly of middle-aged women, is characterized by unilateral disturbance of the facial muscles, resulting in irregular clonic or twitching movements, usually of insidious onset. Mild facial weakness may occur, usually no cause is demonstrated and there is no satisfactory treatment. If exaggerated by emotional reaction, *diazepam* ($\text{Valium}_{GB,US}$) may help. When severe, selective division of branches of the facial nerve or alcohol injection may provide some improvement, though often temporary.

Dental significance

The extent to which dental treatment is practical depends on the severity of the condition.

HENOCH–SCHÖNLEIN PURPURA (ANAPHYLACTOID)

This is a syndrome consisting of purpura, painful joint swelling, abdominal pain, blood in the stools and haematuria. The pathology shows widespread inflammation of small blood vessels with the histological appearance of a hypersensitivity reaction, the precise cause of which is not clear. It occurs mainly in children, frequently following an upper respiratory tract infection. There is no specific treatment. The course is usually benign, lasting 6–8 weeks, but a relapsing course may be seen and 5–10% of patients may develop chronic nephritis.

Dental significance

There is no dental significance.

HEPATITIS

For hepatitis, *see under* Liver disease.

HEPATOLENTICULAR DEGENERATION

For hepatolenticular degeneration, *see under* Liver disease – Cirrhosis.

HEREDITARY HAEMORRHAGIC TELANGIECTASIA (RENDU – OSLER – WEBER SYNDROME)

This is a condition characterized by telangiectases on the face, lips, tongue, fingers, alimentary tract and nasal mucosa. Inheritance is as an autosomal dominant. The lesions increase in number with age and bleeding becomes an increasing problem in adult life with troublesome nosebleeds and gastrointestinal haemorrhage resulting in iron deficiency anaemia. There is no specific treatment besides haemostasis and replacement therapy, although oestrogens may be of value in troublesome epistaxis.

Dental significance

If the telangiectases are present on the lips or in the mouth, care must be taken to avoid damaging them, as haemorrhage may be profuse.

HERPES SIMPLEX (HSV)

There are two antigenic types of the herpes virus hominis. Type I is usually associated with a primary infection of the mouth and type II with infection of the genitals but there can be some cross-over.

Primary herpes

This is an acute infection, usually seen in childhood or adolescence, caused by the herpes virus. The condition is characterized by pyrexia, enlargement of lymph nodes and a crop of vesicles on the gingiva, buccal mucosa, lips and tongue. These rapidly break down to small ulcers and are extremely painful. Vesicles may occur in other parts of the body. Frequently, the condition is seen in patients with immunity disorders or those being treated with immunosuppressants.

Although a large number of treatments have been tried in HSV, at present only *idoxuridine, cytarabine, vidarabine* and *acyclovir* are of importance.

The use of *idoxuridine* in *dimethyl sulphoxide* (DMSO) as a topical application has largely been superseded by topical *acyclovir* (Zovirax cream$_{GB}$), which should be applied five times daily.

For severe primary or recurrent infections systemic treatment is needed. In adults, *acyclovir* is the drug of choice, being less toxic than *cytarabine* – 5 mg/kg given as an infusion over 1 hour every 8 hours. When the mouth is the site affected a *tetracycline* and *amphotericin* mouthwash (Mysteclin$_{GB, US}$) will help to prevent secondary infection. Recovery occurs over about a week.

In children, provided they are able to swallow, treatment is with oral *acyclovir* (Zovirax suspension$_{GB, US}$) 5 ml (200 mg) five times daily for 5 days or half this dose for children under 2 years of age. If unable to swallow and severely ill, they should be admitted to hospital when *acyclovir* can be given by intravenous infusion. *Erythromycin* suspension (Erythroped$_{GB}$, Ilosone$_{GB, US}$) used as a mouthwash four times daily (5 ml containing 125 mg) will prevent secondary infection. It should be held in the mouth as long as possible before being swallowed or spat out.

Recurrent herpes

Recurrent attacks at the same site may occur over a period of years often being precipitated by stress or infection. On the lips and face, where it is known as herpes labialis, topical *acyclovir* (Zovirax cream$_{GB}$), if applied early in the eruption, will hasten resolution. Severe recurrent herpes or recurrences in the immunosuppressed should be treated with systemic *acyclovir* as described for primary herpes.

Dental significance

Children with primary herpes may be brought to the dentist because of the gingivitis, which must be recognized and differentiated from acute ulcerative gingivitis.

By adult life most people have acquired an immunity to the virus and there is no great risk of infection from contact with herpetic patients. However, herpetic whitlows are an occupational hazard of dentists occurring as a result of the virus gaining entry through a small cut on the finger and care should be taken when treating patients with primary or recurrent herpes.

HERPES ZOSTER (SHINGLES)

This condition, caused by the same virus as chickenpox, is due to infection of the posterior root ganglion resulting in severe pain and a vesicular skin eruption in the dermatome supplied by the corresponding posterior root. Occasionally in people with malignant disease or impaired immunity, infection can become generalized and resemble chickenpox. The complications of herpes zoster are more severe in older people. Involvement of the ophthalmic nerve results in corneal lesions which may cause impairment in vision. Geniculate ganglion involvement results in vesicular formation in the pinna over the mastoid and sometimes in the fauces. It can cause facial palsy and loss of taste over the anterior two-thirds of the tongue. Paralysis elsewhere occurs and, although uncommon, encephalitis and myelitis are both described.

Not infrequently, herpes zoster is associated with malignancy and, when occurring in the middle-aged or elderly, without any history of drug treatment, infection or trauma, it should prompt a search for cancer, particularly leukaemia or lymphoma.

Early treatment with steroids may shorten the attack and prevent postherpetic pain but *acyclovir* (Zovirax$_{GB,US}$), a viricidal agent, would now seem the treatment of choice for all but mild cases. A dose of 800 mg should be taken five times daily for 7 days, the dose being spread out over the waking day. However, postherpetic neuralgia often remains a major problem and is extremely difficult to treat. *Carbamazepine* (Tegretol$_{GB,US}$) is the most effective drug with which to treat the condition, but sometimes neurosurgical intervention is required.

Dental significance

When the second and third divisions of the trigeminal nerve are involved the lesions appear on the face and sometimes on the lips and mouth. On the face and lips, 5% *idoxuridine* paint (Herpid$_{GB}$) or 5% *acyclovir* cream (Zovirax cream$_{GB,US}$) should be applied to the lesions four times a day in the prevesicular stage. On the moist surface of the lips and inner cheek, *triamcinolone acetonide* (Adcortyl$_{GB}$, Kenalog$_{US}$) in orobase, will help, while a four times daily mouthwash of *tetracycline* and *amphotericin* (Mysteclin$_{GB,US}$) will help to prevent secondary infection. Usually adults have acquired immunity to the virus in childhood. Thus, although it is possible to develop chickenpox from contact with herpes zoster, in practice this is extremely uncommon. Herpes zoster results from reactivation of previously acquired virus. It does not result from contact either with chickenpox or with herpes zoster. Thus, although a child could contract chickenpox from a dentist suffering from herpes zoster, a dentist would not contract herpes zoster from a patient with either chickenpox or shingles.

HIATUS HERNIA

This is herniation of part of the stomach upwards through the diaphragmatic hiatus into the chest. Herniation may be either sliding or rolling. The former is more common and is the major cause of symptoms which result from acid reflux into the oesophagus which may lead to oesophagitis. However, it should be remembered that sliding hiatus hernias are extremely common and frequently demonstrated on barium meals and the majority give rise to no symptoms even though symptoms are often inappropriately ascribed to them.

Dental significance

If the condition is symptom free with absence of reflux or oesophagitis, no special precautions need be taken. However, if the patient suffers from acid reflux, dental treatment is better carried out without putting the patient into the supine position, and general anaesthetics administered in hospital.

HODGKIN'S DISEASE

For Hodgkin's disease, *see under* Lymphoproliferative disorders – lymphomata.

HUNTINGTON'S DISEASE

For Huntington's disease, *see under* Chorea.

HYDROCEPHALUS

This is an increase in the volume of cerebrospinal fluid (CSF) within the head which may result from an increased production of CSF or interference with its flow or absorption. Hydrocephalus may complicate approximately 2 per 1000 live births. Tumour, infection and subarachnoid haemorrhage may cause hydrocephalus in adults.

Dental significance

Patients with a history of hydrocephalus, which has been treated with an intracranial shunt, will require prophylactic antibiotic cover for dental treatment which is likely to cause a bacteraemia (*see under* Heart disease, infective – Infective endocarditis).

HYPERALDOSTERONISM

For hyperaldosteronism, *see under* Adrenal diseases.

HYPERCHOLESTEROLAEMIA

For hypercholesterolaemia, *see* Hyperlipidaemias.

HYPERGLYCAEMIA

For hyperglycaemia, *see* Diabetes mellitus.

HYPERLIPIDAEMIAS

Frederickson's classification divides these conditions into five types: types I, III and V are rare; type IV is the commonest, accounting for 35–50% of all hyperlipidaemias. The serum is turbid, triglycerides raised, but cholesterol normal. It is associated with obesity and diabetes and the clinical features include xanthomata, lipaemia retinalis and atherosclerosis. Treatment consists of a low-carbohydrate diet. Types IIa and IIb constitute 40% of the cases seen. Here the serum is clear but cholesterol is raised. Xanthomata are present in type IIa but not in type IIb. Both are associated with atherosclerosis and type IIb with diabetes mellitus.

Familial hypercholesterolaemia due to raised low density lipoprotein levels has an autosomal dominant inheritance and is relatively common. The heterozygous form affects between 1 in 300 and 1 in 500 of the population in the UK. The commonent presentation is with early onset of ischaemic heart disease. Fifty per cent of male heterozygotes develop ischaemic heart disease by the age of 50 and presentation at a much younger age is not uncommon. In the homozygous state, the life expectancy is shortened and, until recently, the average life span was 20 years.

Treatment is by dietary modification with a reduction in dietary cholesterol and saturated fats. This may need to be supplemented by bile acid-binding agents such as *cholestyramine* (Questran_{GB}) and lipid-lowering agents such as *bezafibrate* (Bezalip_{GB}) and *atromid* ($\text{Clofibrate}_{GB, US}$).

Dental significance

The association of the condition with diabetes mellitus and ischaemic heart disease should be borne in mind by the dentist. Local anaesthetics without *adrenaline* should be used, and a medical opinion sought before administering a general anaesthetic.

Xanthelasmata on the upper eyelid are often of no significance, but occasionally may be associated with hyperlipidaemia.

HYPERTENSION

Most commonly this is primary or essential where no cause is known, but occasionally hypertension may be secondary to the following diseases: renal disease, Cushing's disease, Conn's syndrome, phaeochromocytoma, renal artery stenosis and coarctation of the aorta.

Mild hypertension may be managed without the use of drugs by reducing salt intake, reduction in weight in those overweight and avoiding high alcohol intake. When drug therapy is required diuretics may provide adequate control, thiazides being the diuretics of choice. For more marked hypertension, there have been major changes in recent years from centrally acting hypotensive agents such as *methyldopa* (Aldomet_{GB}) and *clonidine* (Catapres_{GB}) to the β-adrenoceptor blockers, angiotensin-converting enzyme (ACE) inhibitors and the calcium channel blockers. β-Adrenoceptor blockers work by reducing cardiac output and blocking peripheral adrenoreceptors. All have a hypotensive action, *atenolol* (Tenormin_{GB}) being perhaps the most commonly used. Where control is insufficient a thiazide diuretic may be added. β-Blockers cannot be used in the presence of asthma or heart failure. More recently ACE inhibitors, *captopril* (Capoten_{GB}) and *enalapril* (Innovace_{GB}) have come on to the market for the treatment of hypertension. They are effective and generally well tolerated. As there is little experience of their use long term, they should be used only when β-blockers are not tolerated or are ineffective. Also recently available as hypotensive agents are the calcium channel blockers previously marketed for angina, *nicardipine* (Cardene_{GB}) and *nifedipine* (Adalat_{GB}). Severe hypertension unresponsive to the above drugs or their combinations may require treatment with vasodilator drugs such as *diazoxide* (Endermine_{GB}) or *hydralazine* (Apresoline_{GB}). These are potent drugs, *diazoxide* may cause diabetes and *hydralazine* a systemic lupus erythematosus-like syndrome. The most commonly used hypotensive agents are the β-adrenoceptor blocking drugs of which there are now many on the market. In general, these have fewer side-effects than many of the other hypotensive agents; no one agent seems clearly superior to another. Examples are *atenolol* (Tenormin$_{GB}$) and *metoprolol* (Betaloc$_{GB}$, Lopresor$_{GB, US}$).

Dental significance

There are no contraindications to routine dentistry for patients with hypertension or those taking antihypertensive drugs, provided local anaesthetics with adrenaline are avoided.

Unless the patient is being treated with *warfarin*, blood clotting will be normal, but some increased haemorrhage following dental extractions may be experienced.

Patients recently started on an antihypertensive drug, notably an ACE inhibitor such as *captopril* (Capoten$_{GB}$) or *enalopril* (Innovace$_{GB}$) may experience 'first dose effects' of symptomatic hypotension, and dental treatment is best avoided until this is stabilized.

General anaesthetics in the surgery may be administered to patients with mild hypertension or those in whom the blood pressure is controlled to 180/110 or less, but the blood pressure should be checked immediately prior to administration, immediately afterwards and before the patient leaves. Anaesthetic agents which lower the blood pressure may potentiate the action of antihypertensive drugs, and the patient should remain lying down until the blood pressure has returned to normal, or to its previous level.

HYPOKALAEMIC PERIODIC PARALYSIS

This rare condition, due to episodes of profound hypokalaemia, results in sporadic attacks of muscle weakness or paralysis lasting 1–3 days. The mode of inheritance is mendelian dominant and onset usually in the first or second decade. Rest after excercise, high carbohydrate intake, anxiety and stress may precipitate attacks.

Treatment is by potassium supplements or potassium-retaining diuretics.

Dental significance

There is no dental significance.

IMPETIGO

Impetigo is a skin infection caused by streptococcal or mixed streptococcal and staphylococcal infection. The ostia of the pilosebaceous follicles or sweat ducts are involved, or breaks in the skin due to scratches or bites. It may be associated with scabies or pediculosis. The infection may originate from coccal infections involving the nose, ears or eyes. The typical lesions consist of red raised spots topped with a yellowish-brown crust, most commonly on the face but also on the limbs and in the scalp. The condition frequently occurs in outbreaks affecting several members of the family or school.

Prompt treatment is required as the condition spreads rapidly. Children should be kept away from other children and use a separate towel. *Gentamicin* (Genticin$_{GB}$, Garamycin$_{US}$) cream applied three or four times daily is effective, but if widespread *flucloxacillin* (Floxapen$_{GB}$) 125–250 mg four times daily should be given.

Dental significance

If encountering the condition in a patient, dentists should take care not to pass on the infection via their hands or white coats.

INFARCTION

For infarction, *see under* Heart disease, ischaemic – Myocardial infarction.

INFECTIOUS MONONUCLEOSIS (GLANDULAR FEVER)

This is an acute infectious disease caused by the Epstein–Barr virus (EBV). Although more common in children and adolescents, it occurs in older age groups particularly where there is immunosuppression. It spreads more rapidly under conditions of crowding and close physical contact, being mostly acquired from asymptomatic carriers. Only 6% of cases give a history of contact with the disease. The virus, which cannot be cultured, is said to be present in 10–20%

of routine throat washings. Distribution is worldwide. The incubation period is 30–50 days in adults but shorter, 4–14 days, in young children.

Mild malaise, fatigue and headache may occur during the 4–5 day prodromal phase. Initial clinical symptoms include fever, sore throat and cervical lymphadenopathy. The sore throat may be severe with oedema of the pharynx and exudative tonsillitis lasting several days. Oedema may rarely become severe enough to threaten the airway. In addition to signs in the throat and gland enlargement, splenomegaly commonly occurs and, although hepatomegaly occurs less frequently, liver function tests are frequently abnormal and jaundice is seen in 5% of patients.

Complications include aseptic meningitis, encephalitis, Bell's palsy, thrombocytopenic purpura, haemolytic anaemia, myocarditis and pericarditis.

Diagnosis is confirmed by seeing atypical mononuclear cells in the peripheral blood picture and a positive Paul–Bunnell test. Like the herpes virus, it can become latent and recur if immunity is suppressed, a relapse or prolonged debility being associated with an increased proportion of suppressor T-cells. There is evidence that the Epstein–Barr virus is oncogenic and associated with nasopharyngeal carcinoma and Burkitt's lymphoma.

Treatment is symptomatic. *Prednisolone* may be indicated where pharyngeal oedema is severe, and occasionally tracheotomy is necessary.

Dental significance

Glandular fever should be suspected in children and adolescents who present with an intensely sore throat which is inflamed, oedematous, with small sloughs on the tonsils, and accompanied by fever and cervical adenitis. Less commonly, there are ulcers in the mouth. Antibiotics are ineffective and a sensitivity rash may result from the administration of *ampicillin* ($\text{Amfipen}_{\text{GB}}$, $\text{Penbritin}_{\text{GB}}$).

At this stage the patient is infective and precautions such as face mask for dentist and assistant, and thorough sterilization of instruments and rinse-out glass, should be taken.

INFLUENZA

Influenza is an acute febrile illness of short duration with malaise, fever, generalized aches and pains, headache, often associated with the symptoms of an upper respiratory tract infection. The disease is most commonly caused by influenza viruses A or B. Influenza virus C causes sporadic mild illnes. The incubation period is 2–3 days. The duration of the illness is usually 3–4 days. Influenza may be complicated by encephalomyelitis or secondary bacterial pneumonia.

Prophylactic influenza vaccines have some protective value, lasting up to 1 year, and are best given in November to obtain maximum cover in the danger months. Treatment of the disease is symptomatic. In general the prognosis is good but the infection can cause a high mortality rate among the elderly and those with chronic lung disease. *Amantadine* (Symmetrel$_{GB,US}$) reduces virus shedding and is 80% effective in protecting and treating patients with influenza type A.

By reason of Reye's syndrome occasionally developing in children following infection with influenza A or B, the administration of *aspirin* to children is discouraged.

Dental significance

As a result of their close face-to-face contact with patients, dentists are at risk of picking up 'flu which is spread by droplet infection. There is some doubt about the value of 'flu vaccine as a protection against the endemic disease, but when, as a result of an 'antigen shift', a pandemic breaks out a dentist is well advised to seek vaccine protection. He can, if he wishes, easily administer it to himself and will find clear instructions on the vial. It should not be given to anyone allergic to eggs.

INTRACRANIAL HAEMORRHAGE

Intracranial haemorrhage may result from rupture of veins, as is seen in subdural haematomata, or more commonly arteries, as in subarachnoid haemorrhage. Intracranial haemorrhage may also result from rupture of microaneurysms or cerebral angiomata and extradural haemorrhage from rupture of the meningeal artery.

Extradural haematomata

These result from cranial trauma usually associated with fracture of the temporal bone and consequent rupture of the middle meningeal artery. Typically the patient recovers from the initial trauma only to lapse into unconsciousness with the development of the haematoma. This is a neurosurgical emergency of the first degree, death ensuing unless the bleeding is stopped and the clot evacuated promptly.

Dental significance

Dentists seeing patients with traumatic injuries to the face and jaws must be alert to the possibility of a fracture of the skull occurring at the same time. Any patient who has been knocked unconscious, or who has retrograde amnesia and cannot remember the events leading up to the accident, should be referred to hospital for assessment.

Subdural haematomata

Although occasionally acute, following trauma, most commonly these are chronic resulting from rupture of cortical veins. Although trauma is suspected as a major cause, often there is no history of trauma or the trauma was only mild. Those particularly prone to subdurals are the elderly and those exposed to repeated head trauma such as alcoholics. Diagnosis may be difficult and is often missed. It depends on an awareness of the possibility in the face of vague and varied neurological features, personality change, fits, headaches, and variable level of consciousness. Confirmation comes from computerized tomographic (CT) scan or angiography. Treatment is surgical but, due to the chronic nature of the haematoma, neurological recovery is often disappointing.

Subarachnoid haemorrhage

This is arterial bleeding into the subarachnoid space, usually due to spontaneous rupture of a cerebral aneurysm on the circle of Willis (Berry aneurysm). Symptoms are often dramatic with sudden onset of severe headache sometimes associated with loss of consciousness and followed by meningism and photophobia. One-third of patients die in the first attack, but the prognosis is greatly improved in those who survive the initial 2 weeks.

Treatment is surgical if the aneurysm is accessible.

Intracerebral haemorrhage

When intracranial bleeding occurs within the brain substance, destruction of brain tissue and consequent neurological deficit occurs. Frequency increases with age, predisposing factors being atheroma and hypertension. Onset is sudden, usually with loss of consciousness accompanied by gross neurological deficit. Immediate mortality is high. Treatment of those who survive involves correction of risk factors such as hypertension, careful nursing, and physiotherapy. Permanent neurological damage is usual.

Dental significance

Paralysis and sensory loss may involve the face and mouth, in which case advice and assistance with oral hygiene is required. Wherever possible the natural dentition should be preserved.

IRRITABLE BOWEL SYNDROME (SPASTIC COLON)

This syndrome is characterized by abdominal pain, altered bowel habit, and flatulence and is the commonent cause of patient referral to gastroenterological clinics.

The symptoms result from disordered muscular function of the bowel, in particular the colon, in the absence of disease. The cause is unknown but is thought to relate to the highly refined foods which constitute Western diets.

It is important to exclude organic disease and to reassure the patient to this effect.

Treatment consists of increasing roughage in the diet with bran or other forms of fibre and by the use of smooth muscle relaxants. Response to treatment is unpredictable and often very limited.

Dental significance

There is no dental significance.

ISCHAEMIC COLITIS

For ischaemic colits, *see under* Colitis.

ISCHAEMIC HEART DISEASE

For ischaemic heart disease, *see* Heart disease, ischaemic.

J

JACKSONIAN ATTACKS

For jacksonian attacks, *see* Epilepsy.

JAUNDICE

For jaundice, *see* Biliary disease and Liver disease.

K

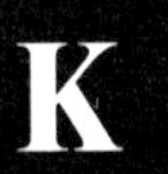

KALA-AZAR

For Kala-azar, *see* Leishmaniasis.

KAPOSI'S SARCOMA

For Kaposi's sarcoma, *see* AIDS.

KAWASAKI SYNDROME

This uncommon disease of children has an incidence of approximately 3 in 100 000, but one which appears to be rising. Its aetiology is unknown, but is probably infective as outbreaks are prone to occur.

Children affected are severely ill with intermittent pyrexia, enlarged lymph nodes and a rash over the whole body. There is a non-purulent conjunctivitis, inflamed throat, strawberry tongue and cracked and bleeding lips. The striking feature is an intense erythema of the palms of the hands and soles of the feet which later desquamate. Some 2% of cases succumb to coronary aneurysms or show some abnormality on the electrocardiogram.

The only helpful treatment to date is with *aspirin*, which poses some dilemma to the physician in view of its association with Reye's syndrome.

Dental significance

Although the dentist is unlikely to encounter a case, it is sensible that he is aware of its existence and the oral manifestations.

KLINEFELTER'S SYNDROME

This is a variety of male hypogonadism characterized by one or more extra X-chromosomes. The condition presents at puberty with gynaecomastia, poor development of secondary sexual characteristics, small testes and eunuchoidal habitus with disproportionately long legs in relation to the trunk. Intellectual impairment of variable degrees is seen.

Dental significance

There is no dental significance.

L

LARYNGITIS

Acute infective laryngitis is usually a complication of a cold, influenza, measles or whooping cough. Besides loss of voice, there is usually a dry cough and, in children, there may be laryngeal oedema and partial respiratory obstruction. Laryngeal oedema can also result from the inhalation of irritants such as steam, chemicals or regurgitated gastric acid.

Treatment of simple laryngitis consists of resting vocal cords as much as possible and avoiding smoking. Inhalations of *tinct. benz. co.* (compound benzoin tincture, friar's balsam), 5 ml to 0.5 litre of boiling water, are usually helpful. Laryngeal oedema requires treatment with *cortisone*, either carried in an aerosol and inhaled such as *betamethasone* (Becotide$_{GB}$) or given systemically. Rarely tracheotomy is required.

Dental significance

Dental treatment should be postponed for patients suffering from laryngitis, and general anaesthetics avoided.

LASSA FEVER

This is one of the viral haemorrhagic fevers (VHF) of Africa, infection occurring as a result of contact with the urine of infected rats or with another patient. It has an incubation period of 21 days and cases are infrequently reported in the UK among those recently returned from Africa. The disease, which is notifiable, carries a high mortality rate, and patients are required to be treated in one of the High Security Infectious Disease Units. Close contacts, which includes those who have had direct contact with patient's blood, are in danger and need to be kept under medical supervision.

Dental significance

In the rare event of hearing that a recently treated patient had subsequently develped Lassa fever, the dentist and assistant should report to the Medical Officer of Environmental Health (MOEH) without delay.

LAURENCE–MOON–BIEDL SYNDROME

This rare familial disorder is characterized by hypogonadism, dwarfism, obesity, mental deficiency, polydactyly and retinitis pigmentosa.

Dental significance

There is no dental significance.

LEGIONNAIRES' DISEASE

An explosive outbreak of fever and pneumonia at an American Legion convention in Philadelphia in 1976 led to the recognition of a previously undescribed group of organisms, *Legionella pneumophila*. Since this time outbreaks and sporadic cases have been described worldwide. Symptoms consist of anorexia, headache, myalgia and fever, associated with diarrhoea, pleurisy, rigors and confusion. Mortality rate is about 10%. Treatment consists of rehydration, oxygen and antibiotics, the most widely used being *erythromycin* ($\text{Erythrocin}_{\text{GB, US}}$) 2–4 g daily. Respiratory support may be necessary.

Dental significance

Although there is no evidence of direct person-to-person infection, the disease is thought to be spread by aerosol inhalation and possibly ingestion. A dentist who learns that he has treated a patient suffering from the condition, should warn waiting-room contacts and patients who have been treated in the surgery immediately after.

LEISHMANIASIS

This disease results from infection by protozoa of the genus *Leishmania*. Infection may be generalized as with *L. donovani* giving rise to visceral leishmaniasis or kala-azar. This has a long incubation period and runs a chronic course with remittent fever, leucopenia and hepatosplenomegaly. Localized infection results from infestation by *L. tropica* causing skin involvement (the oriental sore), or skin and mucous membrane involvement as seen in mucocutaneous leishmaniasis caused by *L. brasiliensis*.

The parasites are all transmitted to man by a species of the sandfly *Phlebotomus*. *Antimonial drugs* are the basis of specific treatment.

Dental significance

In mucocutaneous leishmaniasis, chronic destructive ulcers are found in the mouth and pharynx associated with enlarged cervical lymph glands. To confirm the diagnosis smears or ulcer biopsies are examined for intracellular Leishman–Donovan bodies.

LEPROSY (HANSEN'S DISEASE)

Leprosy is a specific chronic granulomatous disease caused by *Mycobacterium leprae*. It affects the skin, mucosa of the upper respiratory tract and peripheral nerves, causing neuropathic ulceration and muscular atrophy.

It occurs world wide but predominantly in the Tropics. It is not very contagious and the mode of transmission remains poorly understood. Prolonged exposure seems necessary and spread is more likely in crowded conditions with poor hygiene. About 200 new cases are reported each year in the USA and about 20–30 in the UK, almost all in immigrants. Leprosy transmission has not been recorded in England for over 50 years.

Two tissue responses occur:

1. Tuberculoid leprosy with granuloma formation, lymphocyte infiltration and scanty bacilli.
2. Lepromatous leprosy, a destructive lesion teeming with bacilli.

The condition was previously treated with dapsone, but because of the development of dapsone resistance, the WHO study group (1982) designed a single regimen to cover all types of leprosy, treated and untreated, dapsone resistant and dapsone sensitive. It consists of: *rifampicin* 600 mg monthly; *clofazimine* 50 mg daily plus 300 mg monthly; *dapsone* 100 mg daily.

Dental significance

Lepromatous nodules may occur on the lips, tongue and palate, and atrophy of the anterior maxilla may cause loosening of the upper incisors. Involvement of peripheral nerves of the mouth will cause numbness in areas supplied.

LEPTOSPIROSIS

This condition is caused by a Gram-negative aerobic spirochaete, *Leptospira icterohaemorrhagica*, whose hosts are man, rat, dog and cattle, and *L. canicola*, whose hosts are man, dogs and pigs.

Infection is sporadic, classically described in sewage workers and situations where rats occur, but most commonly associated with farming environments. The incidence of the disease is low in the UK. Infection results from environmental contamination by host's urine or by direct contact such as handling infected carcasses.

Clinical presentation may be as a pyrexial illness, an enteric illness, nephritis, aseptic meningitis or as Weil's disease. The incubation period is 7–14 days, the illness lasting 2–14 days.

Onset is often sudden with fever, chills or rigors. There may be headaches, myalgia, arthralgia and often severe prostration. Renal involvement is common but usually minor; less frequently, jaundice and renal failure herald a much more serious form of the disease (Weil's disease). Haemorrhage may be petechial, subconjunctival or massive bleeding with melaena. Haematemesis, haemoptysis and ecchymoses occur. Minor pulmonary involvement is common and myocarditis with dysrhythmias occurs.

Mortality is generally about 10%, recovery usually being complete in those who survive. Treatment is with antibiotics, *penicillin* in high dosage being the drug of choice, together with supportive measures for symptoms and complications.

Dental significance

There is no reported dental significance.

LEUCOPENIA

For leucopenia, *see* Agranulocytosis and neutropenia.

LEUKAEMIA

For leukaemia, *see under* Lymphoproliferative disorders and Myeloproliferative disorders.

LEUKOPLAKIA

Leukoplakia is a negative diagnosis. It is defined by WHO as a white patch which cannot be characterized as any other disease. White patches are found on the gums, tongue and cheeks and are due to thickening and hyperkeratinization of the mucous membrane. The differential diagnosis from atrophic-type lichen planus may not be easy. The condition causes little discomfort, and treatment consists of prohibiting smoking, avoiding hot spiced food and concentrated alcohol.

The problem of leukoplakia is its predisposition to malignant change which appears to be greater when it occurs in certain sites in the mouth and when it is associated with candidal infection.

Dental significance

Opinions differ on the precancerous nature of the condition. The association with malignancy may not be close but, because early detection of it is of such importance, the general practitioner is wise to obtain the opinion of a specialist in all cases of leukoplakia occurring in sites where squamous cell carcinomata of the mouth are found, such as the floor of the mouth and the side of the tongue.

LICE INFECTION

For lice infection, *see* Pediculosis.

LICHEN PLANUS

Lesions appear on the skin as purplish flat patches, and in the mouth as white areas which vary from milk-curd tracery to white plaques and erosions. The condition is more common over the age of 50 and oral and skin lesions occur separately. While the cause is unknown, there are instances where it appears to have been produced by drugs.

Irritation is the main symptom of the skin rash, while in the mouth the lesions are usually symptom free unless erosions are present.

The condition generally resolves on its own, but, if causing discomfort, topical applications of steroids are helpful. On the skin 1% *hydrocortisone* ointment should be applied to the patches, while in the mouth *triamcinolone* dental paste (Adcortyl$_{GB}$, Kenalog$_{US}$) in orobase should be smeared on, or the areas sprayed with *betamethasone* (Becotide$_{GB}$) from an inhaler four times a day after meals.

Dental significance

Malignant change has occasionally occurred in lichen planus of the erosive or atrophic type, and the dentist should carefully note the character and distribution of the condition and reassess at each visit.

LISTERIOSIS

This condition is caused by a Gram-positive bacillus, *Listeria monocytogenes*, found worldwide which infects a wide range of animals. In humans, infection is most commonly intrauterine, the mother having a febrile illness and the baby often premature and dying usually soon after birth. Children may have a septicaemic illness with meningitis. In adults an oculoglandular form is seen with pneumonia and occasionally meningitis.

Penicillin is the treatment of choice. Prognosis is good in the adult form but poor in the infant form unless diagnosis is made early.

Dental significance

No dental significance is known, but one of the authors knows of a dentist who was seriously ill with the infection, but how he contracted it was not discovered.

LIVER DISEASE

Hepatitis

This is a diffuse inflammation of the liver which may result from toxins, drugs or infection. Viral hepatitis is the most common cause and may be subdivided into three main groups.

Hepatitis A

The virus is transmitted by faecal/oral means although blood spread can occur. It is a disease of poor sanitation, overcrowding and institutions, especially those for the mentally handicapped. It is seen commonly in less developed countries, particularly among those travelling to such parts of the world. The virus is present in the blood several days before the liver function tests become abnormal, and disappears with the development of jaundice. The disease is usually self-limiting over a period of weeks but may rarely progress to fulminant hepatic failure. Chronic liver disease does not occur. Serological techniques are now available to confirm infection with the A virus. When travelling abroad to high-risk areas a substantial measure of immunity, lasting 2–3 months, can be obtained by an injection of immune globulin prior to departure. It should not be given within 2 weeks of any live vaccine.

Hepatitis B

Transmission is almost exclusively parenterally, although recent studies have demonstrated faecal/oral transmission. Whole blood or blood fractions passed at transfusions, via surgical or dental instruments, tattoo needles or syringe needles are the commonest routes of infection. However, the virus is found in semen, saliva and urine. The disease is commonest in drug addicts, homosexuals, mentally handicapped individuals and those repeatedly exposed to blood products. The presence of the infection can be confirmed by demonstration of the hepatitis B surface antigen (Australia antigen HBsAg) in serum. This is important, not only in the diagnosis, but also in judging prognosis. In the majority of people the virus is cleared from the blood during recovery following acute illness. In a proportion, the virus persists and often this persistence is associated with the development of chronic liver disease. These people are a continuous hazard to others as they are potentially infectious, particularly if they carry the hepatitis HBe antigen, a polypeptide component of the core of the hepatitis B virus, indicative of active virus replication. However, recent studies using *interferon* (Roferon$_{GB}$) have shown encouraging results in the treatment of persisting hepatitis B antigen positivity.

Delta virus (hepatitis D virus, HDV)

In 1977, a new antigen–antibody system was discovered in the hepatocyte nuclei of HBsAg positive patients. This was called delta. It is a defective virus and dependent on HBsAg for its survival. It is spread by blood or blood products. The combination of delta and hepatitis B infection is associated with severe hepatitis. Delta infection of a hepatitis B carrier usually results in clinical relapse. If hepatitis B is cleared from the blood, delta is also eliminated. Vaccination against hepatitis B protects against delta.

Hepatitis non-A, non-B

This group is probably a heterogeneous group where markers for neither virus A nor virus B are found. It is seen most commonly in those people who develop hepatitis following a transfusion, and in haemophiliacs.

Dental significance

In patients with active hepatitis dental treatment should be postponed until convalescent serological tests reveal the type of virus and whether the patient may still be infective.

Hepatitis A Type A hepatitis presents few risks particular to the dental surgery. The virus disappears from the blood soon after the arrival of jaundice and has not been demonstrated in the saliva.

Hepatitis B (formerly known as Australian antigen positive) In addition to those with active hepatitis, approximately 1 in 1000 of the population of the UK is serologically HBsAg positive, many having no history of the clinical disease. Of these, 1 in 5 is HBeAg positive and the blood and saliva highly infectious. A high proportion of them are to be found among those brought up in less developed countries, drug addicts and homosexuals, Down's syndrome and other mentally handicapped individuals cared for in institutions, those with chronic liver disease, haemophiliacs and those on renal dialysis.

Where possible, dental treatment of patients falling into these categories should be delayed for serological assessments. Those who are HBsAg and HBeAg positive are high-risk patients and should be treated in hospital dental units with special facilities. Included with these must be patients infected with the delta agent, which increases not only the severity of the infection but also its infectivity. Those who are HBsAg positive but anti-HBe are lesser-risk patients and routine dentistry can be carried out in general practice provided special precautions are taken. These include:

1. Face-masks, gloves, and glasses worn by dentist and assistant.
2. Incineration of contaminated material and disposable instruments after use.
3. Efficient autoclave or dry heat sterilization of all instruments.
4. Work surfaces wiped down with disinfectant containing 1% free chlorine or 2% glutaraldehyde.
5. Impressions should either be sent to technicians in sealed bags with a note warning of hepatitis risk, or taken in silicone, washed, and immersed in 2% glutaraldehyde for 4 hours before despatch.

For the last 5 years a vaccine against hepatitis B (H-B-Vax$_{GB}$) has been available in this country. Following three intramuscular injections (in the deltoid muscle for best results) at intervals of 1 and 3 months, 80–90% immunity is conferred on the recipient. Reactions to the vaccine are extremely rare and soreness at the site of injection is of a minor nature. Fears that the agent could be a vector for AIDS were shown to be quite groundless. Recently, a vaccine genetically engineered from yeast has come on the market (Engerix B$_{GB}$). The vaccination routine is as for H-B-Vax$_{GB}$.

The length of time over which immunity is conferred remains a little indefinite. The manufacturers of H-B-Vax$_{GB}$ advise assessment of the antibody titre from a blood sample 5 years after vaccination, and the giving of a booster dose if the antibody level has fallen below 10 IU/l. Levels appear to fall by a factor of 5–10 per year so some idea of how long immunity will last can be gained from the blood investigation.

The Ministry of Health have included dental personnel among

those recommended to receive the vaccine and dentists are foolish if they do not make arrangements for themselves and their dental assistants to be vaccinated; dental students would be well advised to do likewise early on in their studies. Hepatitis B is an extremely unpleasant and occasionally fatal disease, and the implications for a dentist who becomes a chronic carrier are worrying.

Procedure following accidental inoculation in a dentist who has not been vaccinated The blood of patients with active hepatitis and carriers of the disease contains the living virus and will produce the disease if inoculated into another person who is not immune. Modern research indicates that as little as 0.0001 ml of blood from a patient who is HBeAg positive is all that is required, while 1.0 ml of anti-HBeAg blood would probably be safe. The virus can also gain entry through an open cut or blood getting in the eyes. The saliva also contains the virus, but to a lesser extent, and spread by aerosol spray is unlikely. Most dentists cut or pierce their hands from time to time when working on a patient and, if the instrument has been contaminated with blood or saliva, they are at risk. When this occurs, the dentist is advised to make a careful assessment of the risk through questioning the patient and, if he considers it significant, explain the situation and request the patient has a blood test. The nearest laboratory with facilities for this should be contacted by phone and either arrangements made for the patient to visit immediately or a blood sample taken from the patient in the surgery there and then. This is more efficient and less irksome, and only requires the ability of venepuncture and a few sterile syringes, needles and specimen bottles which a local pathology laboratory will usually let you have. The procedure is as follows:

1. With the patient's permission, withdraw 5 ml of venous blood and put it in the specimen bottle avoiding contamination.
2. Cork the bottle securely (the blood will clot in the bottle but this is anticipated), and label with details of patient and investigation required. Seal bottle in a polythene bag and label bag with sticker saying 'Danger of infection' or 'Hepatitis risk'. Put needle and syringe in another plastic bag and arrange for them to be incinerated as soon as possible.
3. Arrange for the specimen to reach the laboratory as soon as possible requesting a result in 36 hours and, if positive, appropriate treatment.
4. Sterilize instruments and disinfect work surfaces and impressions as suggested.

Speed of action is important; the chances of suppressing an attack of hepatitis are much better if hyperimmune γ-globulin is given within 48 hours. Not only is the dentist at risk when dealing with an infected patient, but outbreaks have been traced to dentists carrying the virus. Cuts on the hands should always be covered with waterproof dressings.

Cirrhosis

Cirrhosis is a histological diagnosis based on the development of fibrosis in the liver following parenchymal damage. Aetiological classification is as follows:

1. *Cryptogenic* – commonly no cause for cirrhosis is found.
2. *Cirrhosis* following chronic active hepatitis.
3. *Alcoholic cirrhosis.*
4. *Hepatolenticular degeneration (Wilson's disease)*: this is a rare congenital disorder of copper metabolism inherited as an autosomal recessive. The features of the disease result from the deposition of copper mainly in the brain, liver and kidney due to the deficiency of the copper-carrying protein ceruloplasmin. Damage to the basal ganglia and hepatic cirrhosis result. The importance of the diagnosis is that it is treatable with D-*penicillamine*.
5. *Haemochromatosis*: this is cirrhosis due to massive iron accumulation in the liver, due either to a primary abnormality of iron handling by the body or secondary to multiple blood transfusions. Clinical features are those of cirrhosis together with slate grey discolouration of the skin, testicular atrophy, diabetes mellitus, arthropathy and cardiac failure.

   Diagnosis depends on demonstrating abnormally high serum iron levels and typical biopsy changes.

   Treatment consists of regular venesection and iron chelating agents together with supportive treatment of the complications.
6. *Immunological liver disease–primary biliary cirrhosis.*

Clinical features of cirrhosis

There may be no symptoms or signs in well compensated disease. When symptoms occur they are often vague: dyspepsia, malaise or tiredness. As the cirrhosis progresses features of liver failure occur: jaundice, ascites, mental deterioration, confusion and coma. Haematemesis may occur from bleeding varices.

Diagnosis is confirmed by liver biopsy. Management consists of removing the cause where possible and supportive measures for the complications. Prognosis is very variable but the 5-year survival is approximately 5%, death resulting from liver failure, haemorrhage or hepatoma. Great care should always be taken before the use of any drugs in cirrhotic patients because many are metabolized in the liver and some are hepatotoxic. Cirrhotic patients are particularly sensitive to the effects of sedatives and analgesics.

Dental significance

An unpleasant smell (foetor hepaticus) is often noticeable in the breath of patients suffering from cirrhosis. Symptomless enlargement of the parotid glands has been reported.

Routine dentistry can be undertaken but a reduced synthesis of blood clotting factors often leads to increased haemorrhage following extractions. *Lignocaine* should be used sparingly not more than 4 ml of 0.2% solution at a visit. *Aspirin* and *paracetamol* should be prescribed with caution and narcotic analgesics avoided. All hypnotics and sedatives can precipitate coma and *diazepam* (Valium$_{GB, US}$) should be used in reduced dosage.

Penicillin is safe to prescribe but *chloramphenicol, erythromycin estolate* (Ilisone$_{GB, US}$), *fusidic acid*, and *talampicillin* (Talpen$_{GB}$) are hepatotoxic.

General anaesthetics should be administered in hospital, and halothane avoided as an anaesthetic agent.

LOEFFLER'S SYNDROME

This is a heterogeneous group of lung disorders associated with eosinophilia in the peripheral blood. There are three main types. In all there is abnormal radiological shadowing on the chest X-ray.

1. Pulmonary infiltration with eosinophilia but without asthma. This may result from reaction to parasites such as *Ascaris* sp., to pollens or to drugs. Symptoms are a cough and sometimes fever and malaise.
2. Asthma with eosinophilia. Although eosinophilia is common in asthma, lung shadowing is not and, when present, is most commonly due to added infection with *Aspergillus fumigatus*, which causes a hypersensitivity reaction.
3. Polyarteritis nodosum. This involves the lung in a third of cases, 50% of whom have eosinophilia and asthma.

Dental significance

Asthma when present demands the considerations described under asthma.

LUPUS ERYTHEMATOSUS

For lupus erythematosus, *see* Systemic lupus erythematosus.

LUPUS VULGARIS

This is tuberculous skin involvement usually seen in children, affecting predominantly the face and neck. The skin is scaly, red with telangiectases and the classic 'apple jelly' appearance of individual tubercles when blood is expressed from the lesion with a glass slide. The lesion develops slowly; scarring follows resolution. The bacillus is somewhat attenuated in the skin so *isoniazid* 100 mg three times daily for 6–12 months usually is adequate for curative treatment.

Dental significance

Lesions in the mouth have been reported, but would resolve with systemic treatment given for the skin.

LYELL'S DISEASE

The staphylococcal 'scalded skin syndrome' primarily affects young children. It is caused by an epidermolytic toxin and results in extensive skin erythema and blistering, leading to shedding of sheets of epidermis. Most affected children eventually recover.

Dental significance

The mucosa of the throat and mouth may also be involved.

LYMPHOMATA

For lymphomata, *see under* Lymphoproliferative disorders.

LYMPHOPROLIFERATIVE DISORDERS

These are disorders arising from lymphatic tissue.

Leukaemias

Acute lymphoblastic leukaemia

Bone marrow and blood are infiltrated by the most primitive form of lymphoid cell, the lymphoblast. This leukaemia is more common in children than in adults. Aetiological factors include virus infection and irradiation and the clinical features are anaemia, bleeding and infection. In children the early symptoms are uncharacteristic, including lassitude, irritability and anorexia. Later pyrexia, pallor, enlargement of lymph glands and spleen with pain in the limbs and haemorrhages in the skin and mucous membrane occur.

Treatment with *prednisolone* and *vincristine* (Oncovin$_{GB,US}$) leads to complete remission in 95%, further treatment being required to maintain the remission.

Chronic lymphatic leukaemia

This is a malignant proliferation of lymphocytes, more common in men than in women and more common in the elderly. Fifteen per cent of patients are diagnosed on a routine blood count. Clinical features include lymphadenopathy, malaise, anaemia and splenomegaly. Infection is common due to failure of antibody formation and affects particularly the respiratory system and skin. Haemolytic anaemia and skin infiltration are other complications. The condition does not lead to acute leukaemia. No treatment is indicated in the absence of symptoms. When required, cytotoxic treatment is with *chlorambucil* (Leukeran$_{GB,US}$) or *cyclophosphamide* (Endoxana$_{GB}$, Cytoxan$_{US}$). Corticosteroids are used for thrombocytopenia and haemolytic anaemia, and radiotherapy for glandular masses. Mean survival is 5 years, with 15% surviving to 10 years.

Dental significance

A third of cases of acute lymphatic leukaemia have oral symptoms from the start and may attend for dental advice before the disease has been diagnosed. In chronic lymphocytic leukaemia, oral manifestations tend to occur later.

There is painful swelling of the gingivae associated with infection, bleeding and sloughing of the overlying mucosa. Large ragged ulcers may occur in the mouth and, as a result of the disease or its treatment with immunosuppressants, secondary infection with bacteria or *Candida* sp. is common. Recurrent parotitis is seen but is a rare feature.

Dentists should be alert to the possibility of acute lymphatic leukaemia in the presence of painful gingivitis in the young, and appreciate that the white count may be normal and the examination of a blood film necessary to confirm the diagnosis. In established cases, every assistance should be given to improve oral hygiene and control secondary infection. Mouthwashes and interdental irrigation with 0.2% *chlorhexidine* (Corsodyl$_{GB}$) should be instituted, and candida infection controlled with four times daily use of fungicides, such as *nystatin* (Nystatin Mixture$_{GB}$, Mycostatin oral suspension$_{US}$), *amphotericin* lozenges (Fungilin$_{GB}$), *miconazole* or *ketoconazole*.

A viscous mouthwash containing 2% *lignocaine* or *benzocaine* lozenges 10 mg may be required to ease the discomfort of eating. The prescription of antibiotics should be made in consultation with the physician in charge of treatment.

Lymphomata

Hodgkin's disease

This is a primary disease of lymphoreticular tissue of unknown aetiology, with peak incidence at 25 and 70 years, being more common in men.

Clinical features are painless glandular enlargement, hepato-splenomegaly and bone involvement. Symptoms include pruritus, fever, weakness, malaise, weight loss and anaemia.

Liver involvement leads to jaundice and ascites. Pleural effusions, spinal cord compression, gastrointestinal and skin involvement occur.

Diagnosis depends on biopsy. Radiotherapy is the most effective treatment for localized disease. When generalized, chemotherapy is used.

The following groups of drugs are used, and are sometimes known as the MVPP regimen:

1. Nitrogen mustard: *mustine, chlorambucil* (Leukeran$_{GB,US}$) or *cyclophosphamide* (Endoxana$_{GB}$, Cytoxan$_{US}$).
2. Vinca alkaloids: *vincristine* (Oncovin$_{GB,US}$) and *vinblastine* (Velbe$_{GB}$, Velban$_{US}$).
3. *Procarbazine* (Natulan$_{GB}$, Mutulane$_{US}$).
4. *Prednisolone.*

Overall prognosis is good; 80% of patients go into complete remission and 41% are free of disease at 6 years.

Dental significance

Oral manifestations of Hodgkin's disease are uncommon, and dental problems stem from drugs used in its treatment. Reduced resistance to infection must be expected. Candida infection of the mouth may be controlled with four times daily use of oral fungicides, such as *nystatin* (Nystatin Mixture$_{GB}$, Mycostatin oral suspension$_{US}$) or *amphotericin* lozenges (Fungilin$_{GB}$). Antibiotic cover should be given if extractions are required, and a reduced platelet count may lead to some post-extraction haemorrhage. Previous treatment with steroids should be taken into account (*see* Adrenal insufficiency). General anaesthetics should be given in hospital.

Non-Hodgkin's lymphomata

There are many similarities between Hodgkin's disease and other lymphomata. Clinical presentation and principles of treatment are the same. Burkitt's lymphoma originally described in African children, but more recently reported in Europeans, is a similar condition, but one in which the tumours are more frequently found in the jaw bones.

Dental significance

This is as for Hodgkin's disease.

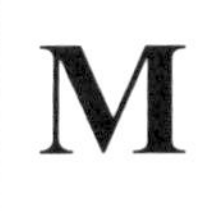

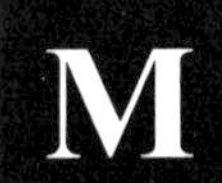

MACROGLOBULINAEMIA (WALDENSTRÖM'S MACROGLOBULINAEMIA)

This is a group of diseases characterized by the presence in the serum of high concentrations of macroglobulin (IgM). It occurs either in isolation or as part of a lymphoproliferative disorder. Clinical features result from hyperviscosity of the blood and include cardiac failure, a bleeding tendency and retinopathy.

Plasmaphaeresis may be life saving, while specific treatment is indicated where lymphoproliferative disease is present.

Dental significance

Bleeding gums and increased post-extraction haemorrhage are the main oral problems of the condition.

The degree of cardiac failure must be considered when dental treatment is required.

MALARIA

This is probably the most widespread disease of developing countries, caused by the protozoan *Plasmodium*. Four species exist: *P. falciparum*, *P. vivax*, *P. malariae* and *P. ovale*. Transmission is by an anopheles mosquito.

Falciparum malaria may be fatal if treatment is delayed, and it is of the greatest importance to consider the diagnosis in any sick person who has returned from an endemic area in the previous 6 months. The clinical features of the different types are:

Malignant tertian malaria (*P. falciparum*)

This has a variable presentation, which includes headaches, malaise, nausea, vomiting, joint pains and fever. Few signs are found and deterioration may be dramatic with drowsiness leading to coma, convulsions and death in 24 hours. Renal failure, hyperpyrexia and massive haemolysis (black water fever) are other features sometimes seen.

Benign tertian (*P. vivax*) and ovale malaria (*P. ovale*)

Fever is the major feature occurring every second day. Splenomegaly and anaemia occur but serious complications are rare.

Quartan malaria (*P. malariae*)

This is similar to benign tertian but fever occurs every 3 days and nephrotic syndrome may occur. Diagnosis depends on identifying the parasite in the blood film.

Chloroquine (Avloclor$_{GB}$, Aralen$_{US}$) cures falciparum malaria without relapse if started in time, because there is no hepatic phase to its life cycle. Treatment of *P. vivax* and *P. ovale* requires additional treatment with *8-aminoquinolone* in order to eradicate the hepatic phase. If uneradicated, relapse of the disease may take place and continue intermittently for 2 or 3 years.

Resistance is increasingly common in south-east Asia, South America and Africa. *Quinine* is the treatment of choice where *chloroquine* resistance is suspected.

Prophylaxis should be taken for a week before entering an endemic area and a month after leaving. One of the following drugs should be used:

proquanil (Paludrine$_{GB}$)	100 mg daily
pyrimethamine (Daraprim$_{GB, US}$)	50 mg weekly
chloroquine (Avloclor$_{GB}$, Aralen$_{US}$)	300 mg weekly

Dental significance

There is no dental significance and no danger of the infection being passed on to the dentist or staff.

MALIGNANCY

Major advances have taken place in recent years in the medical treatment of malignancy. Conditions previously inevitably fatal such as Hodgkin's disease, seminoma and leukaemia may now be cured by radiotherapy, drug therapy or both. In contrast, adenocarcinoma of the gastrointestinal tract remains curable only rarely and then only surgically. Neither radiotherapy nor chemotherapy has made any real impact on these all too common malignancies.

The drugs used in malignancy can be divided into cytotoxic drugs, drugs affecting the immune response, and sex hormones and hormone antagonists such as *tamoxifen*. With increasing survival rates of patients with malignancy and the increasing number of malignancies seen as people live longer, the dentist will be treating an increasing number of patients suffering with malignant disease and on treatment of one kind or another.

Dental significance

Aside from primary malignancy of the oral cavity, which is not within the scope of this book, the dentist should be aware of the influence that malignant disease elsewhere in the body may have on the mouth. Pain related to the tongue, teeth or jaws, oral or facial numbness and weakness of muscles may all result from tumours involving, or exerting pressure on, the fifth and seventh cranial nerves. Occasionally, a metastasis from a tumour elsewhere may be found in the mouth, the commonest site being the gum and the most likely primary a bonchial carcinoma. Patches of pigmentation and bullous formation in the oral mucosa have also been reported in association with malignancy elsewhere in the body. Myelomata and lymphomata may be present in the jaw bones as well as other parts of the body, while infection and bleeding of the gingivae are frequent associations of both myelogenous and lymphatic leukaemia.

Both malignancy itself and the drugs used in its treatment cause debility and suppression of immunity. In the mouth, there is decreased replacement of epithelial cells with progressive thinning of the epithelium, leading to ulceration and sepsis. In the bone marrow, myeloproliferation is reduced with consequent neutropenia and thrombocytopenia. As a result bacterial, fungal and viral infections of the mouth are facilitated and lead to gingivitis, herpes outbreaks and candidiasis.

Preoperative antibiotics should be given if the white blood count is below 1000, and extractions or other surgery avoided if the platelet count is below 50 000. In cooperation with the patient's doctor, *acyclovir* (Zovirax$_{GB, US}$) 200 mg five times daily by mouth may be given to suppress intraoral and labial herpes, while 1 ml *nystatin* (Nystan oral suspension$_{GB}$) (100 000 units) four times daily or 5–10 ml *miconazole* (Daktarin Oral Gel$_{GB}$, Monistat$_{US}$) four times daily should be given for the fungal infection.

MALLORY–WEISS SYNDROME

Gastrointestinal haemorrhage occurs in this syndrome due to laceration of the mucosa at the lower end of the oesophagus following vomiting or retching.

Dental significance

There is no dental significance.

MEASLES

For measles, *see* Morbilli.

MELANOMA

The incidence of this tumour is increasing and is now responsible for 0.8% of all cancers, and 0.6% of cancer deaths. It occurs more in fair-skinned races and may be associated with periodic bouts of sunbathing rather than continuous exposure to sunlight. It seems probable that ultraviolet light is the main aetiological factor. Over half the malignancies arise in a previously recognized mole, lentigo or giant hairy naevus.

Treatment is by surgical excision. Once the lesion has metastasized, response to treatment and prognosis are poor.

Dental significance

In adults a number of malignant melanomata are reported to arise in pre-existing pigmented naevi in the mouth.

MENIÈRE'S DISEASE

This is a chronic disease of the labyrinth characterized by extremely unpleasant attacks of vertigo associated with tinnitus and progressive deafness. Attacks come on suddenly commencing with buzzing, intense vertigo, nausea and vomiting with cerebellar signs on the side of the lesion. Attacks usually last 15 minutes to an hour but may last considerably longer.

Treatment is with sedatives and antihistamines such as *dimenhydrinate* (Dramamine$_{GB, US}$) 50–100 mg three to six times daily, or *prochlorperazine* (Stemetil$_{GB}$, Compazine$_{US}$) 5–25 mg as required up to a maximum of 30 mg in 24 hours. Salt-free diet is said to be beneficial. Surgery is required when medical treatment fails.

Dental significance

Patients generally dislike being placed supine in the dental chair, and treatment in the upright or semi-prone position is more comfortable for them.

MENINGITIS

Bacterial meningitis

Pyogenic bacterial meningitis is most commonly caused by one of three organisms: *Streptococcus pneumoniae* usually seen in adults (a pneumococcus), *Neisseria meningitidis* (a meningococcus) most commonly seen in children and *Haemophilus influenzae* type B also usually seen in children.

Often there is a preceding or concurrent upper respiratory tract infection, ear infection or pneumonia with symptoms of general malaise. Invasion of the meninges by pyogenic organisms is associated with rapid deterioration, high fever, headache and vomiting often followed with 6–24 hours by increasing drowsiness, confusion and coma. With meningococcal infection there may be associated septicaemia, a purpuric rash and occasionally adrenal insufficiency with circulatory collapse. Neck stiffness is not invariable especially in the comatosed patient. Fits are common, especially with infection by *H. influenzae*. Cranial nerve abnormalities may result from involvement of nerves by the inflammatory process. Papilloedema may occur. Examination of the CSF is essential for making the diagnosis, showing a high CSF polymorphonuclear–leucocyte count, a low CSF glucose and bacteria on Gram staining.

Despite early diagnosis and treatment, overall mortality for *H. influenzae* and meningococcal infections remain in the region of 5–10% and may be substantially higher when the diagnosis is delayed. Pneumococcal meningitis carries a higher mortality in the region of 20%. The mortality is highest in neonates and prognosis worse with coma and recurrent fits. Recovery from meningococcal meningitis is usually complete without neurological sequelae, unlike *H. influenzae* or pneumococcal infections which often are associated with mental retardation, fits, hemianopia and blindness.

Successful treatment depends on early diagnosis and appropriate antibiotic therapy. For *Strep. pneumoniae* and *N. meningitidis*, intravenous *benzylpenicillin* is the treatment of choice, while intravenous *chloramphenicol* is the treatment of choice for *H. influenzae*.

Tuberculous meningitis

The frequency of tuberculous meningitis in the community reflects the frequency of tuberculosis in that community. In the UK, tuberculous meningitis is rare. Diagnosis may be difficult and is often delayed. Before antituberculous chemotherapy it was invariably fatal. Initial symptoms may be very non-specific and onset very gradual over some weeks. Headaches and general malaise may later be complicated by fits. Focal cranial nerve lesions are characteristic of the disease. The development of tuberculous endarteritis leads to further neurological damage.

CSF examination reveals a lymphocytosis and a low glucose level.

Treatment is by triple antituberculous therapy using *isoniazid, rifampicin* and *ethambutol.* The average mortality rate is 10% but often permanent neurological damage persists in those who survive.

Viral meningitis

This is the commonest form of meningitis and is usually caused by enteroviruses, especially echovirus and Coxsackie virus. In the UK, mumps virus is the commonest cause of viral meningitis. Often there is some degree of encephalitis associated with the meningitis.

The main clinical features are a fairly rapid onset of headache and neck stiffness, often associated with vomiting, fever and photophobia.

The CSF shows a lymphocytosis but the CSF glucose is not reduced in contrast to bacterial meningitis.

The prognosis is good, the disease is self-limiting and recovery complete.

Dental significance

It is not anticipated that a patient with meningitis will attend for dental treatment, but a dentist might hear of a patient, treated within the last 5 days, who has developed meningococcal meningitis. Under such circumstances, waiting room contacts should be informed and the dentist and dental surgery assistant take the advice of their doctor about prophylactic cover. This is normally recommended only for close contacts and members of the patient's immediate family, *rifampicin* 600 mg every 12 hours for 2 days or *minocycline* 100 mg every 12 hours for 5 days being the antibiotics of choice.

METHAEMOGLOBINAEMIA

This abnormal haemoglobin results either from drug interaction such as with phenacetin and sulphonamides, or with industrial poisons such as dinitrobenzene and aniline dyes. A rare congenital form exists. Cyanosis is the striking clinical feature often in the absence of other symptoms. Treatment involves removal of the cause and large doses of *ascorbic acid.*

Dental significance

There is no dental significance.

MIGRAINE

The presenting symptom is severe headache, accompanied by anorexia, nausea and vomiting may last a few hours or 1–2 days. It is usually preceded by a visual aura and thought to result from an initial arterial constriction followed by vasodilatation. The attacks vary in frequency and may be precipitated by a variety of factors such as anxiety, hormones, various foods or starvation.

Treatment of an attack is with analgesics, usually *aspirin* or *paracetamol*, combined with antinauseants such as *metoclopramide* or *buclizine* (Migravess$_{GB}$, Paramax$_{GB}$, Migraleve$_{GB}$). *Ergotamine* is often helpful and is best given by inhalation (Medihaler-ergotamine$_{GB}$) to obtain rapid absorption.

Prophylactic drugs which are used include *diazepam* (Valium$_{GB,US}$), *propranolol* (Inderal$_{GB,US}$), *clonidine* (Dixarit$_{GB}$), and *methysergide* (Deseril$_{GB}$, Sansert$_{US}$).

Dental significance

Occasionally the pain is experienced in the upper teeth, which can cause dental confusion.

Neither the disease itself nor the drugs used in its treatment are a hazard to dental treatment.

MIKULICZ'S SYNDROME

Enlargement of lacrimal and salivary glands due to lymphoma, lymphocytic anaemia, or sarcoid constitute this syndrome.

Dental significance

With the secretory lobules of the salivary glands being replaced by non-secreting tissue, xerostomia results. Not only will the patient suffer from a dry mouth and loss of taste, but speech and swallowing may be difficult, and the incidence of caries and periodontal disease greatly increased.

Assistance should be given to the patient to maintain oral hygiene, and measures to reduce caries and periodontal breakdown instituted. Daily application of a fluoride gel (Omnigel$_{GB,US}$) and use of *chlorhexidine* (Corsodyl$_{GB}$, Peridex$_{US}$) in an irrigator or as a mouthwash, is advisable. The prescription of an artificial saliva may prove helpful.

This condition is not be be confused with crops of aphthous ulcers, sometimes called Mikulicz's aphthae (ulcers), which are unconnected with the syndrome.

MOLLUSCUM CONTAGIOSUM

This is a papular lesion of the skin caused by a pox virus. The lesion contains a semi-solid caseous material in which masses of virus particles are embedded. The small discrete rounded umbilicated papules most commonly occur on the trunk.

Transmission is by direct contact. The lesion may persist for months or years. Spontaneous resolution occurs. Otherwise treatment can be initiated with podophyllin, salicylic acid, freezing or curettage.

Dental significance

Infection of the mouth has been described but is very unusual.

MONILIASIS

For moniliasis, *see* Candida infection (thrush).

MORBILLI (MEASLES)

This highly infectious fever is caused by a virus and has an incubation period of 10–14 days.

The first manifestations are those of a severe cold with fever, conjunctivitis and sometimes photophia. The mucosa of the mouth is inflamed and small white Koplik's spots are usually visible on the buccal mucosa opposite the molar teeth. The pink/red macular rash appears on the fourth day behind the ears, and spreads to the face and trunk.

The common complications are otitis media and bronchopneumonia, while a rare but serious one is encephalitis.

Although antibiotics are indicated for superadded bacterial infections, there is no evidence that prophylactic antibiotics prevent these complications occurring, and their use is not recommended. In the UK, a single injection of vaccine given at 14 months of age is advised in order to give active immunity. From October 1988, a triple vaccine for measles, mumps and rubella (MMR), given at the same age, will become routine. Mass vaccination has been carried out in the USA for several years and the number of cases of morbilli has been drastically reduced.

Dental significance

The disease is spread by droplet infection, a child being most infectious during the first 5 days. Any contacts in the surgery or waiting room should be warned so they may obtain passive immunity with γ-globulin. Complete suppression may be obtained with a large dose given within 5 days of contact, while a small dose mitigates the condition which still confers active immunity. If measles is severe during early childhood, a band of poor enamel may be seen on the teeth when they erupt.

MOTOR NEURONE DISEASE

This includes amyotrophic lateral sclerosis, progressive muscular atrophy and progressive bulbar palsy. This distressing condition results from degeneration of motor neurones in the anterior horns of the spinal cord and certain cranial nerve nuclei. It occurs mainly in middle age and later.

The commonest presentation is with muscle wasting, starting in the hand muscles and progressing proximally. These muscles characteristically show fasciculation. Cramps and pain occur but there is no sensory loss. Wasting of the upper limbs and spasticity of the legs may occur. A progressive bulbar palsy is seen, especially in women, leading to dysphagia and dysarthria. Wasting and fasciculation of the tongue are characteristic.

The disease progresses unremittingly over approximately 3 years and is invariably fatal. There is no treatment.

Dental significance

The dysphagia which frequently develops with the advance of this distressing disease, makes dental treatment doubly unpleasant. Efficient suction is essential and the extent of dental treatment should be tailored to the patient's physical condition.

MUCOVISCIDOSIS

For mucoviscidosis, *see* Cystic fibrosis.

MULTIPLE ENDOCRINE ADENOMATOSIS

This rare condition, of which three types are recognized, is usually familial and identified by screening families who have a history of the disease. Sporadic cases occur, however, although less commonly in children.

Type I (Wermer's syndrome) is characterized by tumours in the pituitary, pancreas and parathyroid gland.

Type IIa (Sipple's syndrome) is noted for medullary thyroid carcinomata, phaeochromocytomata and hyperparathyroidism.

Type IIb exhibits medullary thyroid carcinoma, phaeochromocytomata, mucosal neuromata and opaque corneal nerves.

Early recognition is important so that medical and surgical treatment can be instituted before it is too late.

Dental significance

Type IIb is commonly associated with a high narrow palate and an orthodontic malocclusion. Multiple sessile mucosal nodules may be found on the tongue, lips and eyelids. Being symptomless they may have not been reported to their doctor by the patient, and the dentist can be the first to notice them. Early referral for investigation may permit treatment before the thyroid carcinoma has spread.

MULTIPLE MYELOMA

For multiple myeloma, *see* Myeloma.

MULTIPLE SCLEROSIS

The cause of this condition remains a mystery – virus infection, deficiency disorders and autoimmune reactions have all been postulated but not proved. It is more common in northern climates and three times more frequent in the Orkneys than in Cornwall. Five to ten per cent of sufferers have relatives with multiple sclerosis and in identical twins the incidence is 20–40%. It may be that an inherent tendency is triggered by a virus.

The demyelination, which characterizes the disease, starts close to a blood vessel, and it is thought that B-lymphocytes may produce antibodies which damage myelin. The demyelinating process occurs at random throughout the nervous system, giving rise to localized motor or sensory loss. It is usual for episodes to be followed by periods of remission which may last several years. In those who contract it in middle age, the condition is more steadily progressive. At the present time there is no effective treatment. *Corticotrophin* (Acthar$_{GB,US}$) may be helpful during episodes of demyelination, and a small multicentre study has shown *amantadine* (Symmetrel$_{GB,US}$) to be of significant benefit in reducing relapses. Hyperbaric oxygen has not stood up to its expectations but diets rich in polyunsaturated fats, such as sunflower oil, are worth keeping to.

Dental significance

While facial numbness is sometimes an early symptom and one which is reported to the dentist, a small number of patients with this condition develop paroxysmal trigeminal neuralgia.

A number of sufferers have the impression that dental extractions, or even a local anaesthetic for conservative work, evoke demyelinating episodes. Though this has not been substantiated, it should be given consideration, the extent of dental treatment being otherwise dictated by the patient's condition and prognosis.

MUMPS

For mumps, *see under* Parotitis – Epidemic parotitis.

MUSCULAR DYSTROPHY

This is a group of genetically determined myopathies.

Duchenne muscular dystrophy

This is a sex-linked recessive disorder almost confined to males, developing between the ages of 1½ and 5 years. All muscles except those of the face are ultimately affected but the proximal lower limb muscles are involved first of all. Cardiac involvement and mental retardation are common. Death occurs before the age of 21.

Facioscapulohumeral muscular dystrophy

The inheritance is dominant and the clinical course very variable in this dystrophy. Childhood development carries a poor prognosis but development is usually in the teens when a benign course is seen. Profound facial weakness with winging of the scapulae later leads to limb muscle involvement.

Limb girdle dystrophy

This rare autosomal recessive disorder has a variable age of onset and initially affects the pelvic girdle causing difficulty in running and climbing stairs. Later the shoulder girdle is involved and severe disability develops by the fourth and fifth decade.

Other dystrophies include Becker type, which is similar to Duchenne dystrophy but more benign, and ocular and oculopharyngeal muscular dystrophy involving extraocular and pharyngeal muscles with droopy eyelids, limited eye movements, limb weakness and dysphagia.

Dental significance

There can be no hard-and-fast rules about the dental treatment of patients with these distressing conditions. The extent and duration of dentistry must be tailored to that which the patient can tolerate, taking into account their life expectancy.

Many suffer from difficulty in swallowing, and treatment must be unhurried and backed up with efficient suction and surgery assistance. General anaesthetics are to be avoided.

MYALGIC ENCEPHALOMYELITIS

For myalgic encephalomyelitis, *see* Benign myalgic encephalomyelitis.

MYASTHENIA GRAVIS

Severe muscle fatigue and muscle weakness are the dominant features of this rare disorder of neuromuscular function. It is seen in all ages and, although more common in women, is considered by biblical historians to be the condition with which Samson was afflicted, being found in men of extraordinary strength and often associated with loss of hair.

Clinical features are muscle weakness of one or more muscle groups, most commonly extraocular and facial, but also bulbar, neck, shoulder and hip muscles. Bulbar and respiratory paralysis may occur. Diagnosis is clinical and confirmed by the response to intravenous *edrophonium chloride*.

Treatment is with anticholinergic drugs, *neostigmine bromide* (Prostigmin$_{GB,US}$) 15 mg three or four times a day or *pyridostigmine* (Mestinon$_{GB,US}$) 60 mg three or four times a day. Intoxication by anticholinergic drugs may lead to a cholinergic crisis, when treatment with assisted ventilation is necessary. *Prednisolone* and immunosuppressive drugs may be valuable in more severe cases. Thymectomy has beneficial results and is now being carried out earlier in the disease.

Dental significance

Patients afflicted may complain of a dry mouth with an increased incidence of caries as a result of inadequate stimulation of the salivary glands. Encouragement and assistance with oral hygiene and caries prevention should be given to those who suffer from the disorder. Dental treatment should be carried out in the mornings, mouth props and efficient suction being helpful to the patient. *Neostigmine* should be taken by the patient 20 minutes before the start of treatment. Local anaesthetics should be administered with caution and *diazepam* (Valium$_{GB, US}$) and *streptomycin* avoided, as they may make the condition worse. General anaesthetics should be avoided, or where essential conducted in hospital.

MYASTHENIC SYNDROME (EATON–LAMBERT)

This condition resembles myasthenia gravis in so far as muscle fatigue occurs, but response to neostigmine is poor or absent and reflexes are usually depressed or missing. It is usually associated with oat-cell carcinoma of the bronchus.

Dental significance

Patients with this condition are unlikely to attend for dental treatment.

MYCOSIS FUNGOIDES

This cutaneous lymphoma is characterized by infiltration of the skin with T-lymphocytes. It begins like a drug eruption or eczema. The lesions become elevated and may spread to peripheral lymph nodes. Ultimately widespread dissemination occurs.

Dental significance

The lesions of this condition are primarily in the skin and only found in the mouth occasionally and then in the terminal stages.

MYELOFIBROSIS

For myelofibrosis, *see under* Myeloproliferative disorders.

MYELOMA

Multiple myeloma is a malignant disease of plasma cells resulting in production of abnormal immunoglobulins from a single clone of cells. This gives rise to a homogeneous immunoglobulin, a paraprotein, or M protein. The condition is rarely seen before the age of 30, affects men more often than women and Negroes more frequently than Caucasians.

Symptoms result from skeletal destruction causing crushed vertebral fractures and bone pain. Disturbance of immunoglobulin leads to infection, and marrow replacement to anaemia and bleeding. Renal failure results from hypercalcaemia and protein deposition in the kidney.

Treatment includes analgesics for pain, the management of complications, anaemia, infection and renal failure, and specific therapy with *melphalan* (Alkeran$_{GB,US}$) or *cyclophosphamide* (Endoxana$_{GB}$, Cytoxan$_{US}$).

Dental significance

Although the incidence of the condition is only 4 in 100 000, the dentist is more likely to encounter a case than carcinoma of the floor of the mouth. Myelomata may develop in the mandible and give rise to pain, resorption of roots and loosening of teeth. Radiologically they appear as round translucent areas. Multiple oozing from the gingiva may follow deep scaling and require treatment with interpapillary injections of local anaesthetic and adrenaline combined with an alginate impression used as a pressure pack. Increased susceptibility to infection and haemorrhage are complications of the disease and should be borne in mind by the dentist treating a case.

MYELOPROLIFERATIVE DISORDERS

Proliferative disorders of the granulocytic, megakaryocytic and erythroid series are known as the myeloproliferative syndrome.

Leukaemia

Acute myelogenous leukaemia (AML)

An accumulation of primitive blast cells is seen in this condition. The aetiology is unknown but might possibly be viral. Clinical features are similar to those of acute lymphoblastic leukaemia: symptoms of anaemia and complications of haemorrhage, infection and tissue infiltration. It occurs more frequently in the middle-aged and elderly than in the young, and is uncommon in childhood. Treatment involves various chemotherapeutic regimens incorporating *cytarabine* (Cytosar$_{GB}$, Cytosar-U$_{US}$), an inhibitor of DNA synthesis, together with supportive care, treatment of anaemia and haemorrhage, and prompt treatment of infection.

Prior to chemotherapy few survived and 50% died within 2 months. Now, at least half of those developing AML achieve complete remission.

Chronic myeloid leukaemia

The onset of this disorder is insidious, occurring more commonly in males and usually between the ages of 20 and 60 years.

Clinical features are weakness, fatigue, malaise, loss of weight and sweating. Splenomegaly and hepatomegaly may cause abdominal discomfort and dyspepsia. Bleeding problems tend to occur later in the disease. Diagnosis is based on a high white cell count, usually greater than 50 000/ml, with myelocytes, metamyelocytes and occasional blast cells. Platelets are often increased in number, the leucocyte alkaline phosphatase is low, and serum vitamin B_{12} level high.

There is a good response to chemotherapy with *busulphan* (Myleran$_{GB,US}$) and remission is easily maintained for 2–3 years. However, sometimes the disease runs a rapid course.

Dental significance

As with lymphatic leukaemias, oral manifestations are worse in the acute disease and may be the presenting symptom. There is painful swelling of the gingivae associated with infection, bleeding and sloughing of the overlying mucosa. Large ragged ulcers may occur in the mouth and, as a result of the disease or its treatment with immunosuppressants, secondary infection with bacteria or *Candida* sp. is common.

Every assistance should be given to improve oral hygiene and control infection. Mouthwashes and interdental irrigation with 0.2% *chlorhexidine* (Corsodyl$_{GB}$, Peridex$_{US}$) should be instituted, and candida infection controlled with four-times-daily use of oral fungicides such as *nystatin* (Nystatin Mixture$_{GB}$, Mycostatin oral suspension$_{US}$), *amphotericin* lozenges (Fungilin$_{GB}$), *miconazole*, or *ketoconazole*. If discomfort is severe 2% viscous *lignocaine* or *benzocaine* lozenges will ease the pain of eating. Dentures should only be worn for meals. The prescription of antibiotics must be made in consultation with the physician in charge of treatment.

Myelofibrosis

In this bone marrow disorder fibrous tissue and sometimes new bone is laid down. In its primary form the cause is unknown, but it may occur secondary to toxic damage to the marrow. The blood picture is of a leuco-erythroblastic anaemia with extramedullary haematopoiesis and hepatosplenomegaly.

Onset is insidious in late middle age with fatigue, weakness and symptoms due to huge splenomegaly and anaemia. The disease runs a prolonged course, infection being a major complication and cause of death. Average survival is 5 years from the time of diagnosis.

Treatment is supportive, androgenic steroids may be beneficial, splenectomy may be indicated for a very large spleen or hypersplenism.

Dental significance

Strict attention to oral hygiene and the control of bacterial and fungal infections of the mouth is important (*see* Leukaemia). Antibiotic cover is essential for extractions.

Polycythaemia rubra vera

This chronic myeloproliferative disorder results in excessive production of red cells causing an increased total red cell mass, packed cell volume and red cell count. The aetiology is unknown. It occurs more commonly in men and in late middle age. Non-specific symptoms include headaches, dizziness, tinnitus and pruritus. Patients have a plethoric appearance. The main features of the disease result from increased blood viscosity and include venous and arterial thromboses, occasionally haemorrhage, ischaemic heart disease and cerebral symptoms with signs of ischaemia and infarction. Splenomegaly increases with the duration of the disease. Treatment is by venesection in the acute phase in combination with ^{32}P or cytotoxic drugs, *chlorambucil* ($\text{Leukeran}_{GB,US}$), *cyclophosphamide* (Endoxana_{GB}, Cytoxan_{US}) or *busulphan* ($\text{Myleran}_{GB,US}$). Without treatment mean survival is 2 years; with venesection mean survival is 4 years, while the combination of venesection and ^{32}P or cytotoxic treatment increases survival to more than 10 years. Early deaths result from thrombosis or haemorrhage, late deaths from marrow failure or leukaemia.

Secondary polycythaemia

As in polycythaemia rubra vera, this condition is associated with increased erythropoietin and an increased red cell mass. It occurs in chronic hypoxic states (i.e. congenital cyanotic heart disease, chronic respiratory failure and exposure to high altitude). It is also seen in association with certain tumours, renal carcinoma, uterine fibroids, cerebellar haemangioblastomata and hepatomata.

Dental significance

The oral mucous membrane is often blue–red in colour with atrophic glossitis and angular cheilitis present.

Post-extraction haemorrhage can be severe, and though blood loss may be beneficial it is better controlled by venesection. When teeth have to be lost they should be extracted one at a time with precautions to arrest bleeding.

Thrombocythaemia

Essential haemorrhagic thrombocythaemia may accompany any of the myeloproliferative syndromes. Patients present with haemorrhagic tendencies because the platelets are abnormal in function as well as number. In addition splenomegaly, moderate leucocytosis, and a high leucocyte alkaline phosphatase are seen.

Prognosis is usually good, although late in the disease lethal forms of myeloproliferative disease may develop.

Treatment is with intermittent ^{32}P.

Dental significance

Bleeding may occur from the gums and submucosal haemorrhages appear on the palate. Extractions should not be undertaken without consultation with the patient's physician.

MYOCARDIAL INFARCTION

For myocardial infarction, *see under* Heart disease, ischaemic.

MYOCARDITIS

Myocarditis is acute damage to heart muscle due to infection, most commonly viral, or toxic agents. Clincal features are a sinus tachycardia, dysrhythmias and occasionally heart failure. Pericarditis may be an additional feature especially when the infective agent is Coxsackie B virus. Non-specific abnormalities are seen on the ECG. Treatment is symptomatic and supportive.

Dental significance

Patients are too ill to attend for dental treatment.

MYOTONICA ATROPHICA

For myotonica atrophica, *see* Dystrophia myotonica.

MYXOEDEMA

For myxoedema, *see* Thyroid disease.

N

NEPHRITIS

For nephritis, *see* Renal disease.

NEPHROTIC SYNDROME

For nephrotic syndrome, *see* Renal disease.

NEUROFIBROMATOSIS

Neurofibromata are benign tumours of the connective tissue sheath and may arise singly on any nerve. They cause no symptoms unless situated where the nerve lies in a bony canal or is constricted by other structures, in which case neuritis and degeneration of the nerve may occur. Developing within the cranium or spinal canal, symptoms from pressure on adjacent nerves will be evident.

Multiple neurofibromata of cutaneous nerves (von Recklinghausen's disease) usually appear in childhood or adolescence. They are frequently associated with areas of skin pigmentation (*café-au-lait* spots) and bone and endocrine disorders (phaeochromocytoma). The tumours form small lumps in the skin varying in size from that of a pea to several centimetres in diameter. In many instances there is a family history of the disorder. There is no treatment other than surgical removal where they are large and unsightly or causing pressure symptoms.

Dental significance

In a few cases the neurofibromata appear in the mouth.

Loss of sensation over the face, eye or mouth will result from pressure on the trigeminal nerve and facial weakness if the seventh nerve is involved.

The possibility of an endocrine disorder should be borne in mind when planning a general anaesthetic.

NEUROSYPHILIS

For neurosyphilis, *see* Syphilis.

NEUTROPENIA

For neutropenia, *see* Agranulocytosis and neutropenia.

O O

OBESITY

Although certain pathological conditions can predispose to excess weight (e.g. hypothyroidism, Cushing's disease and hypothalamic damage), almost invariably no underlying pathology exists. However, simple obesity is seen in families and certain races and, although this may be attributed to environmental influences and eating patterns, it seems probable that an abnormality of fat metabolism exists in some obese subjects.

Obesity is common in affluent society the world over, and constitutes one of the greatest health problems in the Western World. Life expectancy is greatly reduced, as is reflected in insurance premiums for obesity. Other complications include skeletal damage, an increased tendency to diabetes and heart disease. Respiratory complications in extreme obesity, psychiatric disturbances and problems with general anaesthesia and surgery lead to a greatly increased morbidity and mortality rate.

Treatment ranges from dieting to tooth-wiring and bypass gastrointestinal surgery. Response to dieting is often short lived and usually compliance is poor. Intermaxillary tooth wiring is effective and safe but weight tends to be regained once wires are removed due to a resumption of excessive calorie intake. Surgery is hazardous except when performed in centres specializing in such procedures and able to provide careful long-term follow-up.

Dental significance

Gross obesity complicates all dental treatment. Inferior dental nerve blocks are difficult to position accurately and the mass of the cheeks limits access for conservation and surgery.

General anaesthesia is fraught with problems of keeping the airway open if the patient is not intubated, while intubation in itself becomes a more difficult procedure. Wherever possible, local anaesthesia should be used, reinforced with conscious sedation techniques when required.

Fenfluramine (Ponderax$_{GB}$, Pondimin$_{US}$) is a drug frequently prescribed in obesity. Patients taking it may complain of a dry mouth. General anaesthetics should be conducted with caution on patients being treated with this drug, as a fatality has been reported.

Before cooperating in tooth wiring, a dentist should carefully assess the patient's dentition to make sure little permanent damage will result, and carry out conservative and periodontal treatment to render the mouth as healthy as possible. To avoid gingival damage the jaws are best fixed by wires or attachments direct bonded onto the buccal surfaces of the teeth and wired together. Alternatively metal or acrylic cap-splints can be constructed with opposing hooks for wire ligatures. Meticulous instructions to maintain oral hygiene are essential and 0.2% *chlorhexidine* (Corsodyl_{GB}, Peridex_{US}) mouthwash well rinsed between the teeth four times daily, is advisable.

OESOPHAGEAL VARICES

Oesophageal varices result from portal hypertension from whatever cause. In the UK alcoholic liver disease is the most common cause. Massive life-threatening gastrointestinal bleeding is the alarming complication which carries a high mortality.

Surgical treatment by various forms of venous shunts has been almost completely superceded by sclerotherapy – injection of the varices with sclerosant agents via a fibreoptic endoscope.

Dental significance

There is no dental significance.

OESOPHAGITIS

Inflammation of the oesphagus most commonly results from reflux of acid and occasionally bile into the lower oesophagus. It is usually, though not always, associated with the presence of a hiatus hernia.

Symptoms are of heartburn, retrosternal pain, acid reflux and pain which may mimic angina, spreading across the chest and radiating to the neck. Long-standing oesophagitis may be complicated by stricture formation and rarely carcinoma.

Medical treatment is with H_2-receptor antagonists and mucosal coating agents. When this fails in the presence of a hiatus hernia, surgical repair of the hernia may be indicated.

Dental significance

Acid reflux into the oesophagus may result in referred pain being experienced in the throat and molar teeth. Cases have been reported where repeated regurgitation of gastric acid into the mouth has caused enamel erosion of the posterior teeth.

Patients suffering from this condition dislike being treated in the supine position, and the dentist should appreciate their problem and adapt his methods to save them discomfort.

General anaesthetics should be administered in hospital.

OROMANDIBULAR DYSTONIA

This is a movement disorder typified by muscle contraction affecting the mouth, tongue, jaw, larynx and pharynx, resulting in jaw opening and closing and lip protraction or retraction. The lips may be lacerated and the jaw dislocated. Such people are usually unable to cope with dentures. It may occur as part of a generalized torsion dystonia or secondary to drugs, but may appear in isolation in later life.

It is very difficult to control with drugs and is not helped by surgery.

Dental significance

Sadly there is little the dentist can do to help these unfortunate sufferers. Removal of dentures may be necessary to save tongue and cheek biting and the use of a water-resistant cream may help to prevent the lips becoming excoriated through 'mouthing'.

OSTEITIS DEFORMANS (PAGET'S DISEASE)

More common in men than in women, the disease is said to be present in 3% of men over 40, but in most cases is symptomless. In western Europe, its incidence is highest in the UK and lowest in Norway and Sweden. Essentially there is abnormal osteoclastic resorption accompanied by disorderly apposition of new bone. The bones affected in order of frequency are pelvis, lumbosacral spine, skull, tibia, femur and clavicles.

Bone pain, osteoarthrosis and deafness are the usual symptoms. Bending of weight-bearing bones and pathological fracture are common. Sarcoma is luckily rare. The peripheral resistance of the circulation is altered if the disease is widespread and 'high-output' cardiac failure may follow.

There is no cure but *calcitonin* (Calcitare$_{GB}$, Calcimar$_{US}$) injections of 40–160 units daily are helpful. This is a hormone secreted by the parafollicular cells of the thyroid gland and is of porcine or salmon origin. Also used in treatment is *etidronate disodium* (Didronel$_{GB,US}$).

Dental significance

The bones of the jaw are occasionally affected, causing enlargement, spreading of teech and dental anaesthesia. On the radiograph, the lamina dura is missing and the cancellous bone has a ground-glass or cotton-wool appearance. Hypercementosis may be seen on roots of teeth. In the early stages of the disease, characterized by increased vascularity, excessive bleeding follows dental extractions. Later, with bone sclerosis and hypercementosis, extractions become difficult with increased liability to postoperative infection and sequestrae. Enlargement of the dental ridges in the edentulous produces problems with the fit of dentures. Bone demineralization can occur with high doses of *etidronate disodium* and fracture of the jaw is a possibility with difficult extractions.

OSTEITIS FIBROSA CYSTICA

For osteitis fibrosa cystica, *see* Parathyroid disease.

OSTEOARTHRITIS

This very common disorder may be primary where the cause is unknown or secondary to trauma infection or inflammation. It may be associated with certain occupations and with obesity. Frequency increases with age. Joints most commonly affected are the knees, hips, distal interphalangeal joints, and the carpometacarpal joint of the thumb. However almost any joint may be affected, including the temporomandibular joint. Pain and stiffness are gradual in onset and usually absent at rest. Treatment ranges from simple analgesia to anti-inflammatory agents such as *naproxen* (Naprosyn$_{GB, US}$) and *indomethacin* (Indocid$_{GB}$, Indocin$_{US}$) and ultimately surgery where hip replacement has provided some of the most dramatically successful results.

Dental significance

Osteoarthritis of the temporomandibular joint is comparatively uncommon, in the absence of previous trauma. When occurring in the edentulous or those with severe attrition, restoration of correct vertical occlusion is important. Non-steroidal anti-inflammatory drugs such as *naproxen* (Naprosyn$_{GB, US}$) 250 mg twice daily may be helpful, but should not be prescribed for those with a history of peptic ulceration.

OSTEOGENESIS IMPERFECTA

In this disease, characterized by a deficiency of the collagen matrix, the bones are fragile and subject to frequent fracture. In some cases the sclerae of the eyes are blue, the skull enlarged horizontally and hearing impaired through otosclerosis.

There is no treatment but fractures occur less frequently as children grow older.

Dental significance

Dentagenesis imperfecta, with brown or grey dentine, sometimes accompanies the disease. The density of the bone of the mandible is reduced and lower incisors may be fanned forward by the tongue. Mandibular fracture during extractions has not been reported as a hazard.

Patients with osteogenesis imperfecta are said to be more liable to malignant hyperthermia as a result of general anaesthetics, and these should therefore be administered in hospital.

OSTEOMALACIA

The same conditions which produce rickets in the young lead to osteomalacia in the adult, namely dietary deficiency of vitamin D, absorption failure or resistance to its action. It is to be found in the elderly and debilitated, Asian immigrants, and those on anticonvulsant drugs or aluminium hydroxide. It is also associated with renal disease, diseases of the gastrointestinal tract and chronic liver disease.

The mineral content of the bone is depleted with an increase in cancellous bone and osteoid. Bone pain and proximal muscle weakness are common, and pseudo and pathological fractures occur.

Treatment is with *cholecalciferol* or one of the recently synthesized forms of *vitamin D*, the dosage depending on the aetiology of the condition.

Dental significance

The teeth are unaffected but the cortical bone of the jaw and the lamina dura are reduced in thickness, with great liability to fracture. This demands caution when extracting teeth.

OSTEOPETROSIS (ALBERS-SCHÖNBERG DISEASE)

This rare hereditary disease is characterized by increased thickness of cortical bone at the expense of the medulla. 'Marble bones' and 'celery stick' are terms coined to describe their radiographic appearance. Patients suffer from anaemia, compression of cranial nerves and pathological fractures.

There is no treatment.

Dental significance

Abnormal teeth and delayed eruption have been reported when the disease occurs in juveniles. In adults extractions are difficult and should be undertaken with antibiotic cover as a precaution against osteomyelitis.

OSTEOPOROSIS

In this condition, which mainly affects the elderly, there is a general reduction in bone substance, involving both matrix and mineral content. It is seen in women following the menopause, but it is likely that at least a third of us are affected by the condition after the age of 60. Immobilization, hyperthyroidism, rheumatoid arthritis and prolonged steroid administration are predisposing factors. The sequelae are pathological fractures most commonly of the vertebrae, the neck of the femur or the wrist.

Treatment consists of giving *calcium* (Sandocal$_{GB}$) three times daily to produce a calcium intake of 1–1.5 g/day. Oestrogens in women, and androgens in men, may be helpful.

Dental significance

The cortical bone of upper and lower jaws is greatly reduced in thickness and bone trabeculae reduced in number. The maxillary antrum is increased in size and dips down between the roots of the molars. Excessive force during dental extractions can cause fracture of the maxillary tuberosity or the mandible.

Research on the subject in Finland revealed a 40% reduction in fractures in an area where the fluoride level of the drinking water was 1 part per million compared to another area where fluoride was almost absent. So it would appear that water fluoridation can benefit the old as well as the young.

OTITIS

Otitis externa

Inflammation of the external auditory meatus may be acute and painful when resulting from a boil or furuncle in the ear. More commonly it takes the form of a dermatitis or eczema of the meatal skin.

Treatment of the acute bacterial infection is with systemic wide-spectrum antibiotics such as oral *amoxycillin* (Amoxil$_{GB, US}$) 250–500 mg three times daily, while chronic otitis externa is usually treated with topical applications of steroid combined with antimicrobial and fungicidal agents.

Otitis media

Inflammation of the middle ear, is more common in children. Below the age of 4, *Haemophilus influenzae* is the common infective agent, while later a streptococcus is more usual. Pain is acute and there is danger of perforation of the drum if the infection is not brought under control quickly. When the condition is severe an initial dose of *amoxycillin* (Amoxil$_{GB, US}$) should be given by intramuscular injection (125–500 mg according to age) and then 125–500 mg by mouth three times daily. *Trimethoprim* (Monotrim$_{GB}$, Proloprim$_{US}$) either alone or in combination with *sulphamethoxazole* (Bactrim$_{GB}$, Septrin$_{GB}$, Septra$_{US}$) may also be used in treatment of the condition. Chronic otitis media often requires myringotomy and paracentesis with or without insertion of a grommet tube.

Dental significance

Patients with pain originating in the ear sometimes present to the dentist thinking it comes from a back tooth. This should be borne in mind if no dental pathology can be found.

PAGET'S DISEASE

For Paget's disease, *see* Osteitis deformans.

PANCREATIC DISEASE

Pancreatitis

Acute pancreatitis

This condition presents dramatically with severe abdominal pain of sudden onset accompanied by pallor and often shock. It usually necessitates urgent admission to hospital, where it must be differentiated from other abdominal emergencies and acute myocardial infarction. The main aetiological factors are alcohol and gallstones.

Diagnosis is made clinically and supported by very high serum amylase levels.

Treatment commences with immediate resuscitatory measures. Where the patient is shocked, intravenous fluid replacement, avoidance of oral nutrition, nasogastric suction and appropriate analgesia are required. Only in the face of real diagnostic doubt is laparotomy indicated. Pancreatitis may be complicated by diabetes, jaundice, pseudocyst formation, tetany, hypotension and renal failure. Mortality rates in acute pancreatitis are as high as 30%, but those who recover usually do well and few develop relapsing pancreatitis.

Relapsing pancreatitis (acute relapsing)

This uncommon condition, characterized by recurrent attacks of acute pancreatitis, leads to progressive pancreatic damage, pancreatic insufficiency and diabetes.

Chronic pancreatitis

This disorder is characterized by destruction of glandular tissue associated with fibrosis and calcification leading to exocrine and endocrine failure. Unlike acute pancreatitis, biliary disease seems unrelated, but chronic alcoholism may be causative in some people. It does not seem to follow acute pancreatitis. Presentation may be purely with central abdominal pain and no pancreatic insufficiency, or with insufficiency and no pain. Frequently both coexist. Treatment is symptomatic, the constant need for strong painkillers often leading to drug dependency. Insufficiency may be helped by oral *pancreatic enzyme* preparations, and *insulin* may be required to control diabetes.

Dental significance

Coexisting diabetes must always be considered when treating patients with pancreatic disease (*see* Diabetes mellitus). Oral ulceration and irritation of perioral skin has been reported in those taking *pancreatin* in liquid form.

PARALYSIS AGITANS (PARKINSON'S DISEASE)

This common condition of advancing age results from degeneration of the basal ganglia and substantia nigra.

The clinical features are a 'pill-rolling' tremor of the hands, tremor of the legs, jaw and head occurring at rest and diminishing with activity. In addition, increased muscle tone occurs, giving rise to the characteristic 'lead-pipe' rigidity which may take on a 'cogwheel' character when the tremor is present. Postural abnormalities, akinesia giving a mask-like appearance to the face, slowness in initiating movements, mental deterioration, dribbling, and micturition difficulties are common accompanying features. Parkinson's disease may follow encephalitis and parkinsonism results from certain drugs (i.e. *phenothiazines*), but in most cases the aetiology is unknown.

Levodopa is the most powerful available form of treatment and is used in combination with *carbidopa* (Sinemet$_{GB,US}$), an extracerebral decarboxylase inhibitor, or *benserazide* (Madopar$_{GB}$).

For mild symptoms, *amantadine* (Symmetrel$_{GB,US}$) or anticholinergic drugs such as *benzhexol* (Artane$_{GB,US}$) or *orphenadrine* (Disipal$_{GB,US}$) are used.

Dental significance

Tremor may affect the jaw and tongue but does not preclude routine dental treatment. Some difficulty in swallowing is common, and efficient suction is an important adjunct.

Complaints of a dry mouth are frequent with those on treatment with *amantadine* (Symmetrel$_{GB,US}$) and *benzhexol* (Artane$_{GB,US}$). Providing the condition is mild and uncomplicated by other disease, general anaesthetics may be administered at the surgery. Halothane should be avoided in those patients being treated with *levodopa*.

PARATHYROID DISEASE

Hyperparathyroidism

Primary hyperparathyroidism is usually the result of hyperplasia, adenoma or, rarely, carcinoma of a parathyroid gland. The condition is said to be as common as 1 in 1000 in the UK, and is more frequent in women.

It may present on account of renal stone formation with colic, haematuria, renal infection and, occasionally, if diagnosed late, renal failure. Alternatively, it may present with symptoms of hypercalcaemia, anorexia, dyspepsia, weakness, headache, constipation, polyuria and mental changes. A less common presentation is with symptoms of metabolic bone disease, bone pain and pathological fractures. Extensive osteolytic bone changes – most commonly seen in the jaws, tibiae and fingers – are demonstrated radiologically (osteitis fibrosa cystica).

Diagnosis depends on finding a high serum calcium and alkaline phosphatase, a low phosphate and high parathormone level.

Definitive treatment is surgical removal of the affected gland.

Secondary hyperparathyroidism in the response of the parathryoid glands to a low serum calcium, and is seen predominantly in renal disease and malabsorption. Symptoms are of the underlying cause and also of the resultant metabolic bone disease, skeletal pain, proximal muscle weakness, rickets in children, pseudo and pathological fractures. In contrast to primary hyperparathyroidism the serum calcium is low.

Treatment is the correction, where possible, of the underlying disorder and administration of *vitamin D*. This needs to be given in large doses in renal disorders.

Tertiary hyperparathryoidism is a pathological extension of secondary hyperparathyroidism when the gland develops autonomous activity leading to a rise in the serum calcium.

Dental significance

On X-ray there is thinning of the cortical bone, loss of trabeculae and lamina dura, and the appearance of symptomless giant-cell cysts in the bones of the jaw. These only become noticed by the patient if they break through to the surface and present as an epulis.

Not all giant-cell epulides are associated with hyperparathyroidism, but multiple or recurrent ones should alert the dentist to the possibility. Diagnosis is important so that the patient may obtain treatment before irreversible renal damage has occurred.

Hypoparathyroidism

This can occur spontaneously, but more usually results from surgical removal of the parathyroid glands by design or during thyroidectomy. The level of serum calcium falls and tetany with muscle cramps and epileptic fits may occur. In long-standing hypocalcaemia there is a dry scaly skin, brittle nails, and loss of hair.

Treatment is with *calcium* and *vitamin D* in high doses.

Dental significance

Hypoparathyroidism in infants will cause enamel hypoplasia but in the adult no changes in teeth or bones are seen.

PARKINSON'S DISEASE

For Parkinson's disease, *see* Paralysis agitans.

PAROTITIS

Pyogenic parotitis

This is an ascending infection occurring in the debilitated and those with acute specific fevers. It is prevented by attention to oral hygiene and antibiotics.

Epidemic parotitis (mumps)

This is a viral disease, spread by saliva contact or droplet infection, with an incubation period of 3–4 weeks. The painful swelling of the parotid glands is usually bilateral and the orifice of Stensen's duct inflamed. In adolescents and adults, complications are not infrequent and include orchitis, oophoritis, pancreatitis and encephalitis. The only treatment is symptomatic.

Mumps vaccine is given as a preventative measure in the USA, together with rubella and measles vaccine. It is not in general use in the UK, at the present, but there are plans for it to be introduced in the near future.

Dental significance

Children with mumps may be brought to the dentist complaining of pain on eating, and the tender salivary glands need to be distinguished from lymphadenitis resulting from oral infection or tonsillitis. If the condition is suspected, instruments and utensils contaminated with saliva must be carefully sterilized.

Though not completely reliable, serological tests for mumps immunity are available and it would seem sensible that adult dental staff associated with the treatment of children and who have no history of mumps, should have their immune status checked and, if lacking, receive mumps vaccine. Mumps immune globulin is of no help in alleviating symptoms or preventing complications.

A mild form of parotitis has been reported in 1% of children who have received the combined Measles–mumps–rubella (MMR) vaccine 3 weeks previously.

PAROXYSMAL ATRIAL TACHYCARDIA

For paroxysmal atrial tachycardia, *see under* Heart disease, dysrythmias.

PATENT DUCTUS ARTERIOSUS

For patent ductus arteriosus, *see under* Heart disease, congenital.

PEDICULOSIS

The body louse (*Pediculus humanus corporis*), the head louse (*P. humanus* var. *capitis*), and the crab louse (*Phthirus pubis*) are obligatory parasites of man.

The louse has a flat segmented body with six legs. The female lays up to five eggs (nits) a day, which adhere to hair and hatch in about 8 days. The nymphs mature in 14 days and live 4–6 weeks. Lice take two blood meals daily, the bite causing considerable irritation. The body louse attaches to body hair and migrates to clothing where it can survive about a day or, if conditions are cold, up to a week. The head louse attaches to scalp hair. Spread occurs during close contact. Relapsing fever (caused by *Borrelia recurrentis*), typhus and trench fever may be transmitted by lice.

The crab louse attaches to groin and pubic hair and does not usually transmit disease.

Treatment is with *lindane* or *malathion* in shampoo or lotion ($\text{Derbac}_{\text{GB}}$, $\text{Esoderm}_{\text{GB}}$, $\text{Lorexane}_{\text{GB}}$).

Dental significance

Head-to-head and body-to-body contact, or infected clothes, are the usual means of spread, so a dentist is unlikely to pick up the infection from a patient. However, if a head looks as if it might be infected close contact with the patient's hair is best avoided, and the patient advised to seek medical treatment.

PEMPHIGOID

This skin disorder is similar to pemphigus but affects an older age group and may be preceded by urticarial and eczematous reactions. The blisters are large and remain intact longer, being entirely subepidermal. It is an autoimmune disease. Treatment is with systemic steroids.

Dental significance

As in the skin, the bullae in the mouth remain intact for longer than in pemphigus. They are frequently associated with a painful gingivitis.

Treatment is as for pemphigus.

PEMPHIGUS

This rare condition of middle age begins with ulceration of mouth, conjunctiva and, in women, vulva, leading to crops of bullae 0.5–1 cm in diameter which rupture easily leaving a raw bleeding area. The bullae occur within the epidermis. Untreated the condition may be fatal. Like pemphigoid, it is an autoimmune disease.

Treatment is with systemic steroids and azathioprine ($\text{Imuran}_{GB, US}$).

Dental significance

Oral lesions are said to be present in every case of pemphigus and may precede the skin eruption by as much as a year. Bullae break down rapidly in the mouth and the condition presents as superficial ulcers on the buccal mucosa, lips and palate. Discomfort may be marked.

Topical steroids in the form of *hydrocortisone* pellets (Corlan_{GB}) 2.5 mg or *triamcinolone* paste (Adcortyl_{GB}, Kenalog_{US}) or orobase, four times daily will help, but severe cases require *corticosteroids* systemically.

PEPTIC ULCERATION

Peptic ulcers occur in parts of the gastrointestinal tract where acid and pepsin are secreted, most commonly the stomach and first part of duodenum, but occasionally the oesophagus and rarely in Meckel's diverticulum. They are unusual in children but common in adults, occurring in 10% of the population at some stage of their lives. Gastric ulcers occur equally in men and women; duodenal ulcers are three times more common in men. The aetiology remains obscure but acid is an essential ingredient and presumably some defect in the mucosal defence is another.

Pain is the main symptom, usually related to eating and often associated with loss of appetite and nausea.

Modern diagnostic techniques have shown that the traditionally accepted symptomatic differences between gastric and duodenal ulcers do not exist and differentiation can only be made by barium meal or endoscopy.

Major advances in treatment have come with the development of powerful acid lowering H_2-receptor blockers: first *cimetidine* (Tagamet$_{GB,US}$), followed by *ranitidine* (Zantac$_{GB,US}$) and, more recently, *famotidine* (Pepcid$_{GB}$) and *nizatidine* (Axid$_{GB}$). All are equally effective in healing ulcers and in keeping them healed. The newer drugs may have fewer side-effects but are more expensive than *cimetidine*. They are now felt to be safe for long-term maintenance treatment. Another new ulcer healing drug *pirenzepine* (Gastrozepin), a selective anticholinergic drug, acts by inhibiting acid and pepsin secretion. At present it is a second-line treatment.

An alternative approach to ulcer healing is to protect the mucosa rather than reduce acid. Two drugs with this action are available: *tripotassium dicitratobismuthate* (De-Nol$_{GB}$) is a bismuth chelate and binds to the ulcer base; sucralfate (Antepsin$_{GB}$) is a complex of aluminium hydroxide and sulphated sucrose which acts by protecting the ulcer and mucosa from acid and pepsin attack. *Tripotassium dicitratobismuthate* may have an added advantage in being bactericidal to the organism *Campylobacter pylori* which has recently been identified in association with peptic ulceration and may have an aetiological role. This may explain the more prolonged healing that has been demonstrated when ulcers have been healed by *tripotassium dicitratobismuthate*.

More than 30 different antacids are available for symptomatic treatment. Endoscopic examination and biopsy is recommended for all gastric ulcers to exclude carcinoma.

The main complications are haemorrhage, perforation and pyloric stenosis.

Dental significance

Aspirin and *aspirin*-containing analgesics, *diflunisal* (Dolobid$_{GB}$), *mefenamic acid* (Ponstan$_{GB}$, Ponstel$_{US}$) or non-steroidal anti-inflammatory drugs should not be prescribed for patients with peptic ulcers. *Paracetamol* is a safe alternative. For more severe pain, *dextropropoxyphene* (Distalgesic$_{GB}$, Darvon-N$_{US}$) or *dihydrocodeine* (DF118$_{GB}$) may be taken every 4–6 hours.

Delayed gastric emptying may be a feature of the disease, and it is wise to allow an interval of 6 hours between the last meal and a general anaesthetic.

Diazepam (Valium$_{GB, US}$) should be used with caution in those being treated with *cimetidine* (Tagamet$_{GB, US}$) as its action is prolonged.

PERICARDITIS

This is inflammation of the pericardium and may be accompanied by a pericardial effusion.

Acute pericarditis

This may result from infection, most commonly viral, collagen disorders, chemical and metabolic upsets, e.g. uraemia, myocardial infarction and trauma.

Chronic constrictive pericarditis

This frequently follows previous tuberculosis but in many cases no cause is found. Interference with normal heart function leads to circulatory failure.

Treatment of acute pericarditis depends on the cause, and usually consists of supportive therapy.

Where possible surgery is the treatment of choice in chronic constrictive pericarditis.

Dental significance

Patients with acute pericarditis are unlikely to attend for dental treatment, and a past history of the condition poses no contraindications to dentistry unless constrictive pericarditis has developed. In patients with this complication the output of the heart is compromised and general anaesthetics should only be administered in hospital.

PERIODIC FAMILIAL PARALYSIS

For periodic familial paralysis, *see* Familial periodic paralysis.

PERNICIOUS ANAEMIA

For pernicious anaemia, *see* Anaemia.

PERTUSSIS (WHOOPING COUGH)

Pertussis is one of the more distressing infectious fevers of childhood, on occasions leading to permanent lung damage and having a mortality rate of 1 per 1000 among infants under 6 months. There is no maternal conferred immunity, and whooping cough vaccine is seldom offered under 6 months and then only accepted by 60% of the population of the UK at the present time.

The incubation period is 7–14 days, and the illness starts like a chesty cold from which develop the paroxysms of coughing with the characteristic whoop. Treatment with *erythromycin* renders the child non-infectious but does not alleviate the symptoms.

Dental significance

There are no specific points of dental significance but dentists should bear in mind the infectivity of an untreated child and the chance of passing on the infection to another in the waiting room or surgery. Prophylaxis can be obtained by giving *erythromycin* 12.5 mg/kg four times a day for 2 weeks, provided it is started within 6 days of contact.

PETIT MAL

For petit mal, *see under* Epilepsy.

PEUTZ–JEGHERS SYNDROME

Patchy mucocutaneous pigmentation and adenomatous polyps, predominantly of the small intestine, are the main features of this inherited condition. Symptoms result from the polyps and include bouts of abdominal pain, borborygmi, bleeding and symptoms of anaemia. Carcinoma is not a complication of this type of polyposis.

Dental significance

The brown or black patches of pigmentation may occur round the lips and in the mouth.

PHAEOCHROMOCYTOMA

For phaeochromocytoma, *see under* Adrenal diseases.

PHARYNGITIS

Pharyngitis or sore throat is seldom a disease in itself but a prodromal symptom of a cold, influenza or one of the infectious fevers of childhood. The causative agent is frequently a virus and initial treatment with antibiotics not warranted unless accompanying lymphadenitis. An exception is acute epiglottitis, which is more prevalent below the age of 6 and is due to *Haemophilus influenzae* type B. Urgent treatment should be instigated with *ampicillin* 50 mg/kg 6-hourly or *chloramphenicol* 12.5 mg/kg 6-hourly given intravenously if there is any sign of respiratory obstruction.

Dental significance

Where possible dental treatment should be put off for patients suffering from pharyngitis, and general anaesthetics avoided. Surgeon and dental assistants should wear masks to reduce chances of picking up the infection.

PHTHISIS

For phthisis, *see* Tuberculosis.

PIERRE ROBIN SYNDROME

The syndrome, which is evident at birth, is characterized by a midline cleft of the hard and soft palate, mandibular hypoplasia with retrognathos and, as a result of the latter, difficulty in breathing. The tongue falls backwards into the pharynx and causes partial respiratory obstruction. In some instances cardiac defects may be present as well.

Infants so afflicted are best looked after in special baby care units and treatment to relieve the respiratory obstruction and facilitate feeding started immediately.

Dental significance

Suturing the tongue forward, and nursing the infant prone in a special cot, are among the treatment methods advocated, but it has been shown that in experienced hands the fitting of an obturator as soon as possible after birth is both simple and successful. The tongue is held foward, a clear airway maintained and oral feeding soon possible. At a later date the palate is surgically repaired and, in a large number of cases, spontaneous forward growth of the mandible improves the arch discrepancy.

PITYRIASIS ROSEA

The pink or light brown maculopapular rash of this condition is usually symmetrical and frequently follows a single 'herald' patch. It usually affects people between the ages of 10 and 40 and is of unknown aetiology.

Treatment with oral antipruritics or topical corticosteroids may be required if irritation is severe, but there is no specific remedy. In most cases the lesions disappear spontaneously in 6–8 weeks.

Dental significance

There is no dental significance.

PLEURISY

Inflammation of the pleura may occur with or without underlying lung disease, and has many causes. Pulmonary infection and pulmonary infarction due to embolization are the commonest causes but neoplasia, trauma and collagen diseases may be responsible. Clinical features are pain on respiration and a pleural rub on auscultation. In addition, there may be features of the underlying cause, for example, fever, haemoptysis or shortness of breath. In general pleurisy is an indication of underlying disease rather than a disease itself and, therefore, warrants further investigation. Treatment is that of the underlying cause coupled with prescribing of appropriate analgesics.

Dental significance

Emergency treatment to ease pain or preoperative removal of infected teeth is all that will be required in a patient with pleurisy. The question of antibiotic cover should be discussed with the patient's physician. General anaesthetics are best avoided and, if essential, administered in hospital.

PLEURODYNIA

For pleurodynia, *see* Bornholm's disease.

PLUMMER–VINSON SYNDROME

For Plummer–Vinson syndrome, *see under* Anaemia – Iron deficiency anaemia.

PNEUMOCONIOSES (OCCUPATIONAL LUNG DISEASE)

These conditions result from inhalation of inorganic or organic dust in the course of work, leading to a variety of lung disorders, the most common of which are the following.

Anthracosis (coal-workers' pneumoconiosis)

This is due to coal dust and usually causes no symptoms except in 1% when extensive fibrosis occurs (progressive massive fibrosis) giving rise to breathlessness and haemoptysis.

Asbestosis

This condition results from inhaling asbestos particles and is associated with the serious complication of mesothelioma formation.

Silicosis

This results from inhalation of silica-containing dust which causes fibrosis and leads to breathlessness and later haemoptysis.

Dental significance

There are no contraindications to routine dentistry, but general anaesthetics are to be avoided.

PNEUMONIA

This is inflammatory consolidation of the lung and may result from physical or chemical agents. Only infective pneumonias are considered here.

Pneumonias may be classified as primary, occurring in a previously healthy person, or secondary when occurring in association with pre-existing lung disease, influenza, aspiration or immunological impairment. Symptoms are of fever, cough and often pleuritic pain. Classic lobar pneumonia is seldom seen due to the tendency to prescribe antibiotics early.

Lobar pneumonia in a previously healthy person is usually caused by *Streptococcus pneumoniae* and *penicillin* is the antibiotic of choice. In chronic bronchitics and asthmatics pneumonia is likely to be due to *Pneumococcus* sp. or *Haemophilus influenzae*, when *amoxycillin* should be prescribed. Other primary pneumonias, caused by non-bacterial organisms, such as viruses, *Mycoplasma* sp., *Chlamydia* sp. (psittacosis), *Coxiella burnetti* (Q fever), are termed 'primary atypical pneumonias'.

Tetracycline may be effective against several organisms responsible for primary atypical pneumonia.

Dental significance

It is unlikely that a patient suffering from pneumonia will present for dental treatment.

PNEUMOTHORAX

This is the presence of air in the pleural sac, and may be classified as follows: spontaneous pneumothorax, traumatic pneumothorax or tension pneumothorax.

The majority of pneumothoraces are spontaneous and probably result from rupture of small pulmonary bulli, although often no cause is established. Onset is abrupt with chest pain and shortness of breath. Diagnosis is confirmed with a chest X-ray taken in expiration. Recovery may be spontaneous but, with troublesome symptoms and a large degree of lung collapse, a chest drain is advisable to rapidly reflate the lung.

A tension pneumothorax is the most dangerous complication of a pneumothorax. Air accumulates under pressure, collapsing the lung, shifting the mediastinum and causing progressive collapse of the other lung. Without prompt treatment (insertion of a wide-bore needle into the pneumothorax), death ensues.

Traumatic pneumothoraces are seen in association with penetrating chest wounds and may complicate diagnostic or therapeutic needle procedures to the chest.

Pneumothoraces may be recurrent, in which case treatment, either by insertion of irritant material into the pleural cavity or by pleurectomy, is necessary. This is particularly so when pneumothoraces have occurred bilaterally.

Dental significance

Respiration is hampered and vital capacity reduced, so general anaesthetics should be avoided.

POLIOMYELITIS

This is a viral disease with an incubation period of 7–14 days. There are three types of poliovirus and all gain entry through ingested food or water. Once epidemic in the UK, only sporadic cases in non-immunized persons are now recorded.

The disease starts with fever, headache and signs of meningeal irritation, which are followed in a number of cases by asymmetrical paralysis of varying degree.

There is no treatment other than strict rest in the initial stages, and symptomatic treatment of the paralysis later.

Life-long immunity is obtained with either injected polio vaccine (IPV; Salk) or oral polio vaccine (OPV; Sabin). The latter is more commonly used, four to five doses of the oral vaccine being given over the years of childhood and adolescence. Travellers outside Europe, North America and Australasia are well advised to check that they have been immunized.

Two cases have been reported of close relatives of recently immunized children developing an illness similar to poliomyelitis. The relatives had not themselves been previously immunized and it has been suggested that the parental status of children to be immunized should be looked into in this respect.

Dental significance

While recent cases are unlikely to be encountered, the dentist may be called to treat patients with varying degrees of paralysis as a result of poliomyelitis 30 years ago. General dentistry for those in a respirator is quite possible provided adequate suction is available.

POLYARTERITIS NODOSUM

This is a collagen disorder of unknown cause in which focal inflammation of small and medium-sized arteries occurs. It is a multisystem disease, although occasionally it is limited to one organ. In 50% of patients the presenting features are fever, tachycardia, generalized aching, abdominal pain and weight loss. Presentation may be with specific system involvement, for example, asthma, renal failure, neuropathy, coronary artery disease, Raynaud's disease and a variety of skin lesions.

The disease may take a fulminating and rapidly fatal course over weeks or months, or may be extremely mild ending in full recovery. Renal and pulmonary involvement carry a poor prognosis. There is no specific treatment, *corticosteroids* being the mainstay of drug treatment together with supportive treatment for complications.

Dental significance

Oral manifestations seem to be rare although papules in the mouth and oral ulcers have been described. A significant proportion of patients suffering from this condition are hepatitis B antigen positive and routine dental treatment should be undertaken with this in mind (*see under* Liver disease – Hepatitis).

General anaesthetics should be avoided.

POLYCYSTIC DISEASE

For polycystic disease, *see under* Renal disease.

POLYCYTHAEMIA

For polycythaemia, *see under* Myeloproliferative disorders – Polycythaemia rubra vera and Secondary polycythaemia.

POLYMYALGIA RHEUMATICA

This is a muscular rheumatism seen in old people and characterized by pain, stiffness in the neck, shoulders and back, and occasionally low-grade fever. The striking laboratory finding is a greatly raised ESR. It is frequently associated with cranial arteritis. Systemic steroids result in a dramatic response.

Dental significance

Jaw-ache, with tenderness of the masseter and temporal muscles, is a common symptom. Dentists should enquire whether corticosteroids have been taken during the last 12 months and act accordingly (*see* Adrenal insufficiency).

POLYMYOSITIS

For polymyositis, *see* Dermatomyositis.

POLYNEUROPATHY

Simultaneous impairment of multiple peripheral nerves most commonly results in a distal and symmetrical lower motor neurone weakness with disturbance of sensation in some areas. There are many causes:

- Infection:
  - diphtheria
  - leprosy
  - viral
- Metabolic:
  - diabetes
  - uraemia
  - alcohol
  - amyloid
- Poison:
  - heavy metals
  - organic poisons
- Vascular and collagen diseases
- Carcinomata

It is essential to try and establish the underlying cause of the neuropathy, for although with some causes – such as carcinoma and collagen diseases – the changes are likely to be irreversible, in others – such as alcohol, heavy metals and viral – full recovery may occur.

Dental significance

Routine dentistry must be tailored to that which the patient can tolerate. General anaesthetics are inadvisable.

Dentists should appreciate their susceptibility to chronic mercury poisoning and be aware of the clinical picture it produces. The neurological symptoms include tremor of the arms and legs with deterioration of the handwriting, as well as psychic disturbances which are characterized by loss of decision, self-consciousness, timidity and depression. In addition there may be frequent headaches, gingivitis and gastrointestinal symptoms.

Diagnosis is made by analysis of blood and urine levels of mercury.

THE PORPHYRIAS

This is a group of conditions resulting from abnormal porphyrin metabolism. The major groups are erythropoietic and hepatic, based on the anatomical source of the products of porphyrin metabolism.

Erythropoietic porphyrias

The rare congenital form gives rise to severe photosensitivity, with vesicle formation, and subsequent scarring. Deformity of the fingers, hypertrichosis, a pinkish discolouration of the teeth, haemolytic anaemia and splenomegaly are seen.

Erythropoietic protoporphyrin is commoner and causes intense pruritis and burning of the skin, urticaria and weal formation.

Hepatic porphyrias

Some of these are due to a genetic abnormality but in many there is no evidence of this and various toxins are responsible. They may present in one of two ways: either with alimentary, cardiovascular and nervous system symptoms or with symptoms confined to photosensitivity and skin lesions. In acute intermittent porphyria, which is genetically determined, skin manifestations do not occur and symptoms are abdominal pain, motor weakness and paralysis, sensory disturbance, occasionally epilepsy and tachycardia. In porphyria cutanea tarda, cutaneous symptoms predominate with lesions in light-exposed areas, increased pigmentation of skin and hair, and vesicle formation, with secondary infection leading to scarring. The skin is very fragile, minor trauma leading to vesicle formation. Hepatomegaly and jaundice may be seen in some patients, and are often associated with high alcohol intake.

Treatment is preventative, care being taken to avoid precipitating factors. During an attack symptomatic treatment is necessary.

Dental significance

In erythropoietic porphyria the deciduous and permanent teeth have a brown–pink discolouration (erythrodontia) which is fluorescent under ultraviolet light. Periodontal disease is common and the presence of anaemia must be considered if a general anaesthetic is planned.

Hepatic porphyrias carry no oral manifestations, but *barbiturates* are frequently precipitators of intermittent porphyria and should be avoided.

PREGNANCY

Dental significance

Pregnancy gingivitis, which is the main oral manifestation, is thought to result from increased capillary permeability by reason of raised progesterone levels in the blood. It may become evident as early as the second month of pregnancy but quickly diminishes after parturition. Efficient plaque control is important and remains the only treatment.

X-ray examinations during pregnancy should be avoided. Fetal damage is more likely during the early stages of development and all women of child-bearing age should be questioned about the probability of their being pregnant and X-rays postponed if menstruation is overdue.

A year never passes without another drug coming under suspicion of causing fetal abnormalities. To date none used in dentistry has been implicated, but it is a wise precaution to stick to well-tried methods of pain and infection control during this time.

General anaesthetics can be administered to pregnant patients with a few precautions. The third month of pregnancy is best avoided, especially in those with a history of miscarriage, and also the last few weeks when a large gravid uterus can cause respiratory and circulatory embarrassment. A simple blood pressure reading should be taken at the previous appointment and patients in excess of 150/90 referred for a medical opinion prior to administration. Opiates should not be used as premedication, and the anaesthetic should be conducted without any obstruction to the airway, using anaesthetic gases containing 50% oxygen.

During the terminal weeks of pregnancy, partial obstruction of the inferior vena cava from pressure by the uterus can be provoked with the patient in the supine position. Dentists who work on supine patients should appreciate this and allow these patients to sit up from time to time during sessions of conservative or operative dentistry.

PROGRESSIVE MUSCULAR ATROPHY

For progressive muscular atrophy, *see* Muscular dystrophy.

PROSTHETIC HEART VALVES

For prosthetic heart valves, *see under* Heart disease, ischaemic.

PSEUDOMEMBRANOUS COLITIS

For pseudomembranous colitis, *see under* Colitis.

PSITTACOSIS

This is a specific infection of birds caused by an obligate intracellular bacterium *Chlamydia psittaci.* This can be transmitted to man to give an asymptomatic infection, a mild 'flu-like disease, or a serious pneumonic illness with high fever, headache, cough, myalgia and significant mortality.

Tetracycline is the treatment of choice.

Dental significance

There is no dental significance.

PSORIASIS

The cause of this common skin condition is unknown, but it is frequently precipitated by stress or infection and is more common in the winter months. The typical red patches covered with silvery scales can occur anywhere on the body but are more frequent on the knees and elbows. A pustular eruption is also described. Psoriatic arthritis is found in 20% of sufferers and usually affects the joints of the hands and feet.

Treatment is with local application of *coal tar* in a paste or paint, or *dithranol.* Occasionally steroid ointments are recommended. PUVA (psoralen and ultraviolet light) is used when the condition is widespread.

Dental significance

Small white lesions on the gingivae and geographic tongue have been described in patients with psoriasis. Psoriatic arthritis affecting the temporomandibular joint is a recognized but uncommon complication.

PSYCHIATRIC DISORDERS

It is not within the scope of this book to describe psychiatric disease and its treatment. The degree of cooperation for dentistry can only be assessed by enquiries of relatives, doctors and nurses, who are usually helpful in suggesting a line of approach. In the end it falls to the dentist to decide what treatment is advisable and how best it can be carried out. The majority of psychiatric patients present few difficulties, but for a small number dental treatment is only possible after heavy sedation or under anaesthesia.

Almost all patients with psychiatric disorders will be receiving medical treatment and it is important for the dentist to find out the name and dosage of the drugs they are being given. Tricyclic antidepressants, such as *amitriptyline* (Lentizol$_{GB}$, Tryptizol$_{GB}$, Amitil$_{US}$) and *imipramine* (Tofranil$_{GB,US}$) may prevent the uptake of catecholamines and potentiate the action of *adrenaline* and *noradrenaline*. Hence it is wise to avoid using a local anaesthetic with these. Monoamine oxidase inhibitors, such as *phenelzine* (Nardil$_{GB,US}$) and *iproniazid* (Marsilid$_{GB}$) are said to be free of interaction with catecholamines but interact with other sympathomimetic non-catecholamine drugs. However, it is safer to adopt the same routine with local anaesthesia and be careful not to prescribe any preparation containing *amphetamine, ephedrine* or an opiate analgesic, if the patient has been on these drugs within the last 14 days. *Phenytoin* (Epanutin$_{GB}$, Dilantin$_{US}$) is sometimes given for psychiatric disorders. Its effect on the gums is a problem (*see* Epilepsy) and it is known to potentiate the action of *diazepam* (Valium$_{GB,US}$).

PULMONARY EMBOLISM

For pulmonary embolism, *see under* Embolism – Pulmonary emboli.

PYELONEPHRITIS

For pyelonephritis, *see under* Renal disease.

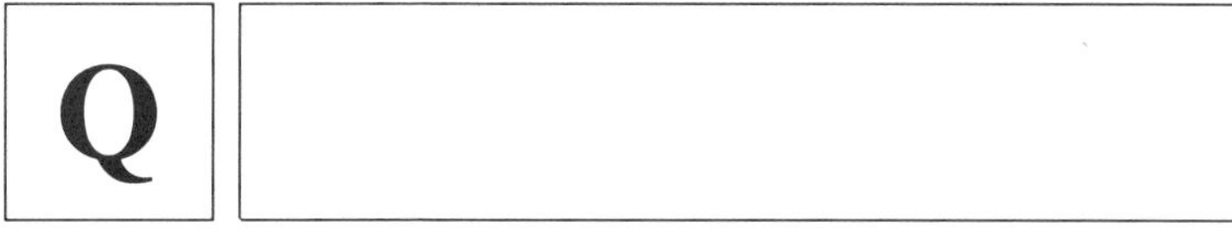
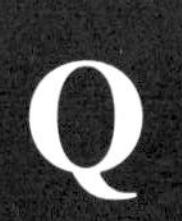

Q FEVER

For Q fever, *see Coxiella burnetti.*

QUINSY

For quinsy, *see* Tonsillitis.

R

R

RAMSAY HUNT SYNDROME

For Ramsay Hunt syndrome, *see* Bell's palsy.

RAYNAUD'S PHENOMENON

The features of Raynaud's phenomenon are intermittent pallor and cyanosis of the extremities brought on by cold or emotion, with return to normal colour between attacks. Trauma, hormones or cigarette smoke may also provoke an attack. Raynaud's phenomenon may occur as an isolated phenomenon, usually with no long-term sequelae. However, it complicates conditions such as scleroderma, systemic lupus erythematosus and polyarteritis nodosum, when the prognosis is less favourable and related to that of the associated disease.

Treatment includes protection from cold and wet, and the use of α-adrenergic blocking agents and calcium antagonists such as *phenoxybenzamine* (Dibenyline$_{GB}$, Dibenzyline$_{US}$) and *nifedipine* (Adalat$_{GB, US}$) and, when medical management fails, sympathectomy.

Dental significance

Delayed healing of extraction sockets has been reported, and it should be appreciated that gum hyperplasia is sometimes associated with the use of *nifedipine*.

REITER'S SYNDROME

This condition, which is sexually transmitted and causes inflammation of the urethra, conjunctivae and joints, occurs predominantly in males, most commonly between the ages of 20 and 30. The three parts of the body become involved in the order mentioned, with a 3- or 4-day interval before spreading to the next. The causative agent is unknown. There is no effective treatment, but the condition usually resolves on its own.

Dental significance

Oral lesions in the form of small elevated red spots or vesicles occur in approximately 25% of cases. They are seen on the gums and buccal mucosa and are usually painless. Involvement of the temporomandibular joint with the arthritis is rare.

Although there is no record of this condition being transmitted other than sexually and the causative organism remains obscure, it would seem sensible to observe high levels of disinfection if a case is seen in the surgery.

RENAL DISEASE

Glomerulonephritis

The clinical presentation of glomerular disease is extremely variable, the main features being proteinuria, haematuria and hypertension. The following syndromes are recognized modes of presentation: acute nephritis, nephrotic syndrome, asymptomatic proteinuria, recurrent haematuria, hypertension, and acute and chronic renal failure.

Definitive diagnosis depends on renal biopsy. Glomerulonephritis may be primary or secondary to underlying disease, such as systemic lupus erythematosus, diabetes and amyloid. The commoner and clinically more important types are the following.

Membranous glomerulonephritis

Diffuse uniform thickening of the glomerular capillary wall is the histological feature of this type of glomerulonephritis. It usually presents as the nephrotic syndrome, the features of which are hypoalbuminaemia, gross proteinuria, hypercholesterolaemia and oedema. It may complicate certain infections – malaria, hepatitis B and syphilis – and may result from certain drugs, penicillamine and gold. Other conditions, such as Hodgkin's disease, carcinoma of breast, sarcoid and diabetes mellitus, may also give rise to membranous glomerulonephritis, but frequently no cause is established.

Management includes a high-protein, low-sodium diet, diuretic therapy and regular follow-up.

Minimal lesion glomerulonephritis

This syndrome is characterized by severe proteinuria and only minimal abnormality on renal biopsy. It occurs in children and its cause is not known. It runs a relapsing course and carries a good prognosis, spontaneous remission occurring in 30%. Treatment includes diuretic therapy and systemic steroids.

Diffuse proliferative glomerulonephritis

The hallmark of this condition is an increase in the number of cells in the glomerular tuft. Presentation is extremely variable but usually takes the form of an acute nephritis, or, occasionally, nephrotic syndrome. It may occur at any age with no sex preponderance. The majority of cases are thought to be due to deposition of small, soluble, circulating immune complexes in glomerular capillary walls as seen in poststreptococcal glomerulonephritis.

Poststreptococcal glomerulonephritis

This type of proliferative glomerulonephritis develops as a result of immune complex formation following streptococcal infection, usually in children of school age.

Clinical features are frequently those of an acute nephritis with oliguria, haematuria, hypertension and impaired renal function. Full recovery occurs in 80–90% but a few have persisting minor renal abnormalities and death occasionally occurs in the acute phase. Management involves treatment of the acute infection, control of hypertension, close observation of renal function and long-term follow-up.

Focal glomerulonephritis

As its name implies, this is a patchy disease of the glomeruli, frequently associated with systemic diseases such as systemic lupus erythematosus, Henoch–Schönlein purpura, and subacute bacterial endocarditis. It presents with haematuria and sometimes acute nephritis or nephrotic syndrome. Clinical features are extremely variable. The cause is not known but the prognosis is usually good.

Pyelonephritis

Chronic pyelonephritis is a common cause of renal failure, occurring more often in women than in men. It may occur as a primary event or secondary to functional or anatomical renal abnormalities. Intestinal bacteria, *Escherichia coli*, *Proteus vulgaris* and *Pseudomonas* sp., are the commonest causes of infection. The condition may be asymptomatic or give rise to frequency and dysuria. In an acute attack malaise, fever, rigors, vomiting and headache dominate the picture, together with marked renal tenderness on examination. Preventative treatment is important as there is no cure for established chronic pyelonephritis. Personal hygiene, prompt treatment of infection and exclusion of anatomical abnormalities when recurrent urinary infections occur, are all important.

Polycystic disease

This relatively common inherited condition which is inherited as an autosomal dominant is characterized by bilateral renal cyst formation and usually presents with renal impairment in the third or fourth decade. Clinical features include abdominal pain, increase in girth, haematuria, hypertension and renal colic. It is one of the four commonest causes of chronic renal failure in the UK in the 30–50 age groups.

Dialysis and transplantation are usually offered to those patients and have favourable results.

Acute renal failure

Prerenal, renal and postrenal factors can lead to acute renal failure. Hypovolaemia from saline depletion, haemorrhage or burns are the major prerenal cause and, with prompt treatment, the prognosis is good. Renal causes include nephrotoxins, renal ischaemia, septicaemia, acute glomerulonephritis, and arterial and venous thromboses. Obstructions to urine outflow from whatever cause will lead ultimately to postrenal failure. The clinical features of renal failure result from electrolyte and fluid disturbances, and are anorexia, nausea, vomiting, dyspnoea, circulatory overload, drowsiness, confusion, occasionally convulsions and coma. Secondary infection is a major hazard.

Treatment depends on the cause. Once renal failure is established management should be in an intensive care unit, special attention being given to fluid balance, electrolyte intake, acid–base balance, nutrition and prevention of infection. Dialysis will be necessary when there is a high blood urea, high blood potassium, fluid overload or severe metabolic acidosis.

Chronic renal failure

The major causes of chronic renal failure in Europe are glomerulonephritis (48%), pyelonephritis (20%) and cystic disease of the kidney (8%). Symptoms are multiple and varied and include fatigue, dyspnoea, anorexia, nausea, vomiting, diarrhoea, bleeding and, occasionally, fits.

Once diagnosed, careful consideration must be given to the control of hypertension, intercurrent illness, gastrointestinal upsets and avoiding nephrotoxic drugs.

Suitability of patients for eventual haemodialysis or transplantation should be considered early on. Management consists initially of control by dietary measures. Ultimately dialysis will be necessary; indications include fluid overload, hyperkalaemia, pericarditis, neurological complications and increasing malaise.

Dental significance

Disease of the kidneys produces no signs in the mouth until renal failure sets in. With acute renal failure, a dry brown-furred tongue is to be found, accompanied by gingival haemorrhages, while in the chronic condition exudative stomatitis, oral ulcers and keratosis may be seen. The oral features improve with successful treatment of the general condition, but in the meantime advice and assistance with oral hygiene is important, together with local treatment of candidal or bacterial mouth infection.

It must be appreciated that there is frequently an electrolyte imbalance, anaemia of varying degree, prolonged bleeding and clotting time and delayed excretion of drugs. Some drugs are nephrotoxic and should not be given to patients with renal disease. They include *tetracycline*, which may cause the blood urea to rise when glomerular filtration rate is reduced, *talampicillin* (Talpen$_{GB}$), *cephaloridine* (Ceporex$_{GB}$, Loridine$_{US}$) and aminoglycosides such as *gentamicin*. Hypnotics, sedatives and tranquilizers should be prescribed with caution as their action may be extended. *Penicillin, ampicillin* and *erythromycin* are safe but *metronidazole* (Flagyl$_{GB, US}$) should be prescribed in reduced dosage. *Aspirin*, *diflunisal* (Dolobid$_{GB}$) and non-steroidal anti-inflammatory drugs are best avoided, but *paracetamol/acetaminophen* (Panadol$_{GB}$, Tylenol$_{US}$) is safe to use. Concurrent or previous treatment with steroids demands special precautions (*see* Adrenal insufficiency *under* Adrenal diseases – Addison's disease).

Renal dialysis patients carry a risk of being hepatitis B antigen positive. Dental treatment for them is best carried out on the day after dialysis. Children on dialysis may suffer from enamel hypoplasia but their caries rate is low. Exposed pulps should not be capped but efficiently root-filled. It would be thoughtful if dentists enquired of dialysis patients which arm the shunt is in and made sure it is comfortable. Patients scheduled for a kidney transplant will be on *azathioprine* (Imuran$_{GB, US}$) and steroids for the rest of their lives. If possible, all dentistry should be completed beforehand and all efforts made to maintain a high standard of oral hygiene.

RENDU–OSLER–WEBER SYNDROME

For Rendu–Osler–Weber syndrome, *see* Hereditary haemorrhagic telangiectasia.

REYE'S SYNDROME

This is a rare, but sometimes fatal condition affecting children during the course of a viral infection.

The clinical picture of persistent vomiting of sudden onset shortly followed by a change in conscious level, results from an encephalopathy complicated by hepatic dysfunction. Its incidence is less than 1 per 100 000, with equal sex distribution, but it is more common in rural areas. In the USA, the median age is 8–9 years but, in the UK, it is 14 months. The precise aetiology is unknown but, in a number of cases, a link with aspirin has been observed.

Dental significance

Aspirin should be avoided in children and young adolescents, *paracetamol/acetaminophen* being given as a mild analgesic, when required.

RHEUMATIC FEVER

This inflammatory disease results from pharyngeal infection with a group A streptococcus. It occurs most commonly between the ages of 5 and 15 years in approximately 3% of those with exudative streptococcal pharyngitis. Those who have had rheumatic fever are more likely to have further attacks than the general population. The disease is multisystem, affecting heart, joints, central nervous system, skin and subcutaneous tissue. Clinical manifestations are fever, migratory polyarthritis and carditis, but Sydenham's chorea, subcutaneous nodules and erythema marginatum are common features. Although joint symptoms may dominate the clinical picture, the serious sequelae relate to valvular and myocardial heart damage, death occasionally occurring in the acute phase.

Treatment in the acute phase is with intramuscular *procaine penicillin* (0.6 g daily), given to eliminate the streptococcus, while symptomatic treatment is given for arthralgia. Preventative treatment is important, especially in those with a history of rheumatic fever who should have long-term prophylactic *penicillin* (0.2 g twice daily) or *sulphadiazine* (1 g daily). All patients under 18 years should receive such treatment. Over 18 years of age the duration of treatment is debatable but 5 years is recommended. Prevention of the initial rheumatic attack depends on prompt vigorous treatment of group A streptococcal infections.

Dental significance

Antibiotic cover is required for any dental procedure likely to cause a bacteraemia in patients who may be suffering from rheumatic fever or whose heart valves may have been damaged by the disease in the past (*see under* Heart disease, infective – Infective endocarditis).

General anaesthetics should not be given without an assessment by a physician.

RHEUMATOID ARTHRITIS

The cause of this chronic systemic disease is unknown. Its main feature is a symmetrical inflammatory arthritis which may be accompanied by haematological, pulmonary, neurological and cardiovascular manifestations. The peak age of onset is in the fourth decade and a genetic predisposition is suggested by the association with the histocompatibility antigen HLA-DW4. Onset is usually insidious, fatigue, weakness, stiffness and myalgia preceding the development of joint swelling. The proximal interphalangeal, metacarpophalangeal, wrist, knee, elbow and ankle joints are most commonly involved. Atlantoaxial joint involvement may result in instability of the upper cervical spine. Temporomandibular joint involvement may interfere with mastication and pain may be referred to the middle ear and throat.

A diffuse interstitial fibrosis may affect the lungs. Heart disease is uncommon but amyloid may complicate the condition, leading to renal failure.

There is an association between rheumatoid arthritis, splenomegaly and leucopenia, termed 'Felty's syndrome'. Other features of this syndrome may include normocytic normochromic anaemia, thrombocytopenia, lymphadenopathy and cutaneous pigmentation. The main hazard is recurrent infection. The syndrome is usually found in patients with severe nodular erosive disease and other extra-articular features.

Ten to twenty per cent of patients have a complete remission or mild intermittent disease while 10% progress inexorably to crippling arthritis. Careful continuous medical supervision is essential, aiming to maintain the patient's ability to function as normally as possible. The objects of treatment are to reduce inflammation and pain, maintain motion and strength, and prevent joint deformity by appropriate physiotherapy, anti-inflammatory drugs, splints, physical rest and orthopaedic surgery. Drug therapy includes the use of *aspirin*, NSAIDs, steroids, *penicillamine* and gold.

Dental significance

The temporomandibular joint is affected in over 50% of patients suffering from this disease. Apart from general treatment, sufferers may be helped by the fitting of a soft bite-raising appliance, carefully constructed to keep the posterior teeth apart by about 3 mm.

Anaemia, either iron deficiency or the anaemia of chronic disorders, frequently accompanies this disease and should be borne in mind if multiple extractions are contemplated. Antibiotic cover must be considered if there is leucopenia.

Sjögren's syndrome of xerostomia and conjunctivitis sicca, with or without enlargement of the salivary and lacrimal glands, sometimes accompanies the condition.

Small ulcers on the buccal mucosa and tongue and an unpleasant taste in the mouth may be seen in patients whose arthritis is being treated with gold salts or *penicillamine*. Those on cytotoxic immunosuppressants may suffer extensive mucosal breakdown and gingival haemorrhages.

Recent treatment with steroids must be taken into account when extractions or anaesthetics are being planned (*see* Adrenal insufficiency *under* Adrenal diseases – Addison's disease).

Patients on non-steroidal anti-inflammatory drugs should not be prescribed *aspirin*.

Antibiotic cover for dental procedures likely to cause a bacteraemia, as described under Heart disease, infective-Infective endocarditis, should be given to patients with artificial joints.

RICKETS

For rickets, *see under* Vitamin deficiencies – Vitamin D.

RINGWORM

For ringworm, *see* Tinea.

ROYAL FREE DISEASE

For Royal Free disease, *see* Benign myalgic encephalomyelitis.

RUBELLA (GERMAN MEASLES)

Rubella is a mild infectious fever with an incubation period of 2–3 weeks. Its characteristics are a rash of pink macules which remain discrete, and enlargement of the occipital lymph nodes.

The danger of rubella lies in the high incidence of fetal abnormality if it is contracted during the first 4 months of pregnancy. For those who have not had rubella in childhood, immunity can be obtained from vaccination with a single dose of attenuated rubella virus. It must not be given if already pregnant.

Dental significance

By reason of frequent close contact with children there is an occupational hazard of rubella in dentistry. All non-immune female dentists and surgery staff should be vaccinated. In the event of pregnant non-immune personnel coming in contact with the disease, high-titre immunoglobulin should be given as soon as possible.

SALIVARY CALCULI

Salivary calculi are three times more common in the submandibular gland and its duct than in the other salivary glands. They cause pain on eating and their presence is frequently complicated by infection of the gland. Near the orifice of the duct they can be localized by palpation, while more distally an X-ray (angled to avoid superimposition of the mandible) will be required to disclose their presence. Stones in the duct can usually be removed by intraoral surgery but if situated in the substance of the gland the submandibular gland must be removed via an external approach.

Dental significance

Small stones impacted near the duct orifice can be removed by the dentist quite simply with a small infiltration of local anaesthetic. After clamping the duct distally to stop them slipping back the duct is incised over them and they are eased out.

SARCOIDOSIS

This is a multisystem granulomatous disorder of unknown aetiology commonly affecting young adults and presenting most frequently with bilateral hilar lymphadenopathy, pulmonary infiltration and skin and eye lesions. Other organs commonly involved are peripheral lymph nodes, liver, spleen, parotids, muscle, heart, mucous membrane and nervous system.

The clinical picture is very variable.

Diagnosis may be incidental on a routine chest X-ray or the disease may present with severe incapacitating symptoms, including fever, weight loss, fatigue and general malaise. Dyspnoea accompanies pulmonary involvement; uveitis and keratoconjunctivitis sicca are features of eye involvement. Skin lesions occur in 30% of patients and include erythema nodosum, erythematous raised infiltrated lesions or non-specific papules or plaques. Variable neurological lesions include isolated facial weakness, peripheral neuropathy and disordered swallowing.

Diagnosis is made on the clinical features and may be supported by histology and a positive Kveim reaction. No treatment may be necessary but steroids are the treatment of choice with progressive pulmonary disease, active ocular disease, central nervous system involvement, hypercalcaemia, myocardial disease and persistent systemic illness. In general the prognosis for sarcoid is good, 80–85% recovering from the disease. Occasionally, patients die from cardiac or renal involvement but, in the majority, the outcome depends on pulmonary involvement where, in a small percentage, plumonary fibrosis is progressive and disabling.

Dental significance

Dark red sarcoid nodules are sometimes found on the palate or elsewhere in the mouth. They are painless and seldom ulcerate. As with other diseases treated with steroids, special precautions must be taken when extractions or general anaesthetics are planned (*see* Adrenal insufficiency). If pulmonary fibrosis has developed, general anaesthetics should be conducted in hospital.

SCABIES

The disease is caused by infection with a mite (*Sarcoptes*), picked up by close body contact or through infected clothes or bedding. The short burrows of the female mite can be found in the epidermis of the limbs and trunk but seldom on the head and neck. Itching is intense and hence secondary infection is common as a result of scratching.

Treatment consists of thorough overall cleaning, followed by two applications of *benzyl benzoate* (Ascabiol$_{GB}$) or *gamma benzene hydrochloride* (Quellada$_{GB}$). Residual irritation may continue for several days. Clothing and bedding should be thoroughly washed.

Dental significance

The burrows being uncommon on the head and neck, it is most unlikely that a dentist will pick up scabies from an infected patient.

SCARLET FEVER

This disorder results from streptococcal production of erythrogenic toxin. The infection is usually pharyngeal and the rash develops within 2 days, spreading to involve the whole body, sparing the palms and soles. Punctate erythema and petechiae occur on the soft palate. The tongue is coated initially but this is shed to leave the typical raw 'red raspberry tongue'. The rash lasts 4–5 days and is followed by extensive desquamation.

Dental significance

There is no dental significance.

SCLERODERMA

For scleroderma, *see* Systemic sclerosis.

SCURVY

For scurvy, *see under* Vitamin deficiencies – Vitamin C.

SHINGLES

For shingles, *see* Herpes zoster.

SICKLE-CELL ANAEMIA

For sickle-cell anaemia, *see under* Anaemia – Haemolytic anaemias.

SILICOSIS

For silicosis, *see under* Pneumoconioses.

SINUSITIS

Infection of the maxillary and frontal sinuses usually follows a cold. Initially the agent is a virus but secondary bacterial infection follows. Pain is felt over the sinus involved, and with infection of the frontal sinus there may be swelling above the eye.

Treatment is with inhalations of *tinct. benz. co.* (friar's balsam) 5 ml in 500 ml of hot water, and decongestant nose drops run in to reach the ostium of the sinus involved. Examples of these are *ephedrine* nose drops, *oxymetazoline* (Alfrazine$_{GB}$, Iliadinene$_{GB}$, Alfrin$_{US}$), and *xylometazoline* (Otrivine$_{GB}$, Otrivin$_{US}$), but they should not be prescribed for patients on treatment with monoamine oxidase inhibitors or antihypertensive agents. Antibiotics are required for frontal sinusitis and maxillary sinusitis which does not respond to these measures.

Chronic sinusitis requires operative treatment.

Dental significance

Because of the proximity of the maxillary sinus to the apices of the upper premolar and molar teeth, patients with sinusitis may visit the dentist complaining of toothache. The recent history of a cold with persistent nasal congestion should alert the dentist to the possible cause of their discomfort.

SJÖGREN'S SYNDROME

This condition occurs predominantly in females of middle age and is caused by lymphocyte infiltration of the lacrimal and salivary glands greatly reducing their natural secretions. It is frequently associated with rheumatoid arthritis and other connective tissue diseases. Patients complain of prickly inflamed eyes, dysphagia and a dry mouth and, on examination, the tongue is found to be dry, shiny and fissured and there may be oral ulceration and candidal infection.

Local treatment consists of keeping the eyes and mouth lubricated with drops and mouthwashes containing 1 or 2% *methylcellulose*, *glycerin* lozenges and lemon sweets to encourage saliva flow. Immunosuppressive agents and corticosteroids may help but are usually reserved for severe cases. Malignant lymphoma is a complication.

Dental significance

In those with teeth an increase in caries is an inevitable sequel, and advice and assistance with oral hygiene is important. The edentulous will experience difficulty in keeping dentures in place.

STEVENS–JOHNSON SYNDROME

This is a severe form of erythema multiforme with development of extensive exudative, bullous and erosive cutaneous lesions involving the mouth, conjunctivae, cornea and genitals. Pannus formation and blindness may result. Fever, vomiting and polyarthralgia may occur. Like erythema multiforme, it is found as a reaction to an infection, of which herpes is the most common, or to drugs such as *penicillin*, *sulphonamides* or *barbiturates*.

The condition is extremely distressing and urgent treatment with systemic steroids is required to prevent serious ocular complications.

Dental significance

The lesions may occur anywhere in the mouth but are seen with greatest regularity on the lips. They start as vesicles which rapidly coalesce and break down to large painful ulcers whose base is covered by a slough or pseudomembrane. On the lips haemorrhagic crusting will be seen. Treatment is with *hydrocortisone* in the form of 1% ointment on the lips and as 2.5 mg lozenges (Corlan$_{GB}$) or *triamcinolone* paste (Adcortyl$_{GB}$, Kenalog$_{US}$) in orobase in the mouth. *Chlorhexidine* (Corsodyl$_{GB}$, Peridex$_{US}$) 0.2% mouthwash will help to prevent secondary infection.

STOKES–ADAMS ATTACKS

For Stokes–Adams attacks, *see under* Heart disease, dysrhythmias.

STROKE

For stroke, *see under* Vascular disease.

SUBACUTE BACTERIAL ENDOCARDITIS

For subacute bacterial endocarditis, *see under* Heart disease, infective – Infective endocarditis.

SUBACUTE COMBINED DEGENERATION OF THE CORD

This is the most serious consequence of deficiency of vitamin B_{12} and occurs in association with pernicious anaemia. The white matter of the spinal cord degenerates leading to progressive irreversible damage to the posterior and lateral columns and there is an associated peripheral neuropathy.

First symptoms are usually numbness or tingling of the feet, leading to unsteadiness on walking and progressive weakness. Examination reveals weakness, loss of vibration and position sense, absent knee and ankle reflexes, and extensor plantar responses. Romberg's sign is positive. Untreated the condition progresses to paralysis. Optic atrophy and mental changes are a feature in a few people. It is essential to be aware of this complication of vitamin B_{12} deficiency and to treat promptly with intramuscular injections of *hydroxocobalamin* (1000 mg on alternate days for a month then monthly permanently) before irreversible neurological damage occurs.

Dental significance

The manifestations of the condition should be borne in mind when a patient presents with glossitis and recurrent oral ulceration. These painful symptoms may lead a patient to take advice while neglecting the early neurological features of the disease.

SUBARACHNOID HAEMORRHAGE

For subarachnoid haemorrhage, *see under* Intracranial haemorrhage.

SYDENHAM'S CHOREA

For Sydenham's chorea, *see under* Chorea.

SYNCOPE

This is a brief, transient and totally reversible loss of consciousness due to acute arterial hypotension. The most common form is vasovagal syncope (fainting) when the patient is usually in the upright position, feels 'faint', and becomes pale, sweaty and tachypnoeic. The syncope is accompanied by a bradycardia and hypotension. Recovery is rapid in the recumbent position.

Dental significance

There must be few dentists who have not experienced vasovagal syncope in a patient before or after a local anaesthetic injection. The immediate treatment is to lay the patient flat and recovery is rapid. The danger of the condition is when it is unnoticed and the patient restrained in the upright position with resulting cerebral anoxia. There is strong evidence to show that several deaths have occurred under anaesthesia in an upright dental chair from this cause. The authors believe that general dental anaesthetics should only be given to patients in the supine position and that those who have just had a local anaesthetic injection should not be left unattended.

SYPHILIS

Syphilis is now less common than other venereal diseases but remains an important medical problem. It results from infection by the spirochaete *Treponema pallidum*. Incubation ranges from 9 to 90 days. The primary lesion develops from a macule to a papule and eventually to an ulcer (chancre) which is painless and usually on the genitals but occasionally extragenital, on the lips, tongue, fingers, nipples or anus. Secondary syphilis develops within 6–8 weeks of the primary sore and is a generalized non-irritant dull red rash. There may follow a symptomless stage (latent syphilis) prior to development of late or tertiary syphilis. Late syphilis may occur within 5 years of the primary sore or may appear much later, when involvement of the skin, cardiovascular system, central nervous system or skeleton may occur. The late lesion or gumma may affect the skin, various viscera and mucous membranes. The tibia is the commonest bone involved. Aortitis may lead to aortic aneurysm formation and aortic incompetence. Neurosyphilis may give rise to meningovascular involvement with headaches, cranial nerve involvement and cerebrovascular accidents due to arterial involvement. Spinal column involvement causes tabes dorsalis with impaired proprioception and vibration sense, muscular hypotonia, Argyll Robertson pupils, ataxia, lightning pains in the legs, and transient severe abdominal pain. Generalized cortical involvement leads to general paralysis of the insane (GPI). Diagnosis is made clinically and confirmed in the early stages by demonstrating the spirochaete, and in all stages by serological tests [Venereal Disease Reference Laboratory (VDRL), fluorescent treponemal antibody (FTA) and *Treponema pallidum* immobilization (TPI) tests].

The patient with late syphilis is no longer infectious.

Penicillin is the mainstay of treatment (daily intramuscular *procaine penicillin* 1–2 g for 10 days in the early stages of acquired infection). For late syphilis 20 g are given in 3 weeks. Results in neurosyphilis are variable, good in meningovascular disease, unpredictable in GPI and poor in tabes dorsalis.

Dental significance

Although tertiary syphilis is less common, the dentist may still meet the condition in the primary or secondary stage.

A primary chancre on the lips or tongue presents as a round or oval ulcer 1–2 cm across with a red indurated base. Unless secondarily infected it causes little pain, but is always accompanied by enlargement of the regional lymph nodes. In secondary syphilis raised grey–white patches are to be seen on the fauces, tongue and palate, which break down and coalesce to form the snail-track ulcer. The lymph nodes are enlarged. Both the stages are infectious to the dentist and subsequent patients. If suspicious, avoid examining the lesions with unprotected hands and make sure all instruments and utensils are effectively sterilized.

In tertiary syphilis gummata are sometimes found on the palate and tongue and are distinguished by their characteristic punched-out appearance. Chronic glossitis and leukoplakia are other oral manifestations of this stage.

SYRINGOMYELIA

This uncommon condition results from cavitation in the brain stem and spinal cord, possibly relating to a congenital abnormality. Dissociated sensory loss with preserved sensation to touch but loss of pain and temperature sensation is characteristic. Muscular atrophy occurs predominantly in the upper limbs. Surgery can halt progression so early diagnosis is important.

Dental significance

There may be loss of pain and thermal sensation over the distribution of the trigeminal nerve with weakness of the palate and tongue if the cavitation extends into the brain stem.

SYSTEMPIC LUPUS ERYTHEMATOSUS (SLE)

This multisystem disorder occurs predominantly in young women and is characterized by many non-organ-specific antibodies. As might be expected clinical features are protean and depend on the particular system most affected. They include the characteristic facial 'butterfly' rash, discoid skin lesions, Raynaud's phenomenon, arthritis, pleurisy, pericarditis, psychoses and nephritis.

Laboratory findings include a normochromic anaemia, positive direct Coombs' test, leucopenia and thrombocytopenia.

The diagnosis is made clinically but supported by the presence of LE cells and antinuclear antibodies, and confirmed by antibodies to double-stranded DNA.

Treatment is largely symptomatic and supportive. Steroids, antimalarials and immunosuppressive drugs have been beneficial in some patients.

Dental significance

Erythematous patches may be found on the buccal mucosa and gingivae, frequently bilateral, like the butterfly rash on the face. When the disease is widespread, anaemia, leucopenia and thrombocytopenia should be taken into account and extractions carried out under antibiotic cover, anticipating increased post-extraction haemorrhage.

Previous steroid treatment may have depressed the adrenals (*see* Adrenal insufficiency *under* Adrenal diseases – Addison's disease).

General anaesthetics should be avoided where cardiac and pulmonary complications exist.

SYSTEMIC SCLEROSIS

Progressive systemic sclerosis is a disorder of connective tissue leading to fibrosis of the skin (scleroderma) and various internal organs, notably the gastrointestinal tract, lungs, heart and kidneys. Its cause is unknown.

The onset is insidious, often with Raynaud's phenomenon, then symmetrical swelling and stiffening of the fingers. The skin becomes tight, firm and bound to underlying subcutaneous tissue.

The hands, arms, face and upper trunk are mainly involved. The facial features appear pinched and the mouth tight and narrowed. Gastrointestinal involvement leads to reflux oesophagitis, dysphagia and malabsorption. Cough and dyspnoea herald pulmonary involvement. Cardiac dysrhythmias and various degrees of heart block indicate cardiac involvement. Renal failure is the main cause of death.

The CRST syndrome is a variant of scleroderma characterized by calcinosis, Raynaud's phenomenon, sclerodactyly and telangiectasia, but without visceral involvement except for the oesophagus.

Diagnosis is clinical. There is no specific treatment and most patients pursue a progressive downhill course.

Dental significance

Reduced facial movement and a mask-like expression results from fibrosis in the skin of the face. The lips lose mobility, being either drawn back from the anterior teeth or 'pursed' due to circumoral constriction. The tongue loses mobility and patients suffer from difficulty in feeding and swallowing. There is an increase in caries and periodontal disease. Limited mouth opening adds difficulties to routine dentistry, and dryness of the mouth and fibrosis may cause problems with the wearing of dentures. Advice and assistance with oral hygiene is of great importance.

General anaesthetics are to be avoided.

TEMPORAL ARTERITIS

For temporal arteritis, *see* Giant cell arteritis.

TETANUS

The causative organism is *Clostridium tetani*, the spores of which are to be found in soil, dust, clothing and the intestinal tract of animals and man. They enter the body with penetrating wounds. Because of the strict anaerobic conditions needed for growth, tetanus is fortunately rare despite the ubiquity of the organism.

After an incubation period varying from a few days to 2–3 weeks the commonest early symptoms are trismus and pain with stiffness in the neck, back and abdomen. In moderate and severe cases generalized muscle spasm with opisthotonus and cyanosis develop within 24 hours.

Special tetanus units are equipped for treatment, which includes large doses of antitoxin, antibiotics to prevent pulmonary infection, and scoline and general anaesthesia to control the spasms. The survival rate is only 50%.

Prophylaxis should be given to all infants in the form of triple vaccine during their first year with one or two boosters in later childhood. For an immunized person a further dose of toxoid should be given following a susceptible injury, while a person not immunized will require 250–500 units of human antitetanus immunoglobulin.

Dental significance

Soil- and dirt-contaminated wounds of the face and mouth may be an entry portal for the organism, and it is the duty of dentists to check the immunity of a patient and act accordingly.

TETANY

This is a syndrome manifested by flexor spasm at the wrist and ankle (carpopedal spasm), muscle twitching and cramps resulting from low serum calcium or metabolic or respiratory alkalosis.

Dental significance

There is no dental significance.

THALASSAEMIA

For thalassaemia, *see under* Anaemia – Haemolytic anaemias.

THROMBOCYTHAEMIA

For thrombocythaemia, *see under* Myeloproliferative disorders.

THROMBOCYTOPENIA

There are many causes of a low platelet count. Spontaneous bleeding is uncommon if the platelet count is the only abnormality unless the count falls to very low levels, 20 000/mm^3 or less. A relatively low platelet count is, however, of significance when surgical procedures are envisaged.

Low counts result from either failure of platelet production, for example marrow aplasia and neoplastic involvement of the bone marrow, or from reduction which may occur due to drug sensitivity, disseminated intravascular coagulation, systemic lupus erythematosus, massive blood transfusion and hypersplenism.

Dental significance

Small submucosal haemorrhages are frequently found on the palate and there may be bleeding from the gingivae.

There should be consultation with a view to platelet transfusion before extractions are undertaken.

THRUSH

For thrush, *see* Candida infection.

THYROID DISEASE

Hyperthyroidism

The two common causes of hyperthyroidism are evident where the gland is diffusely enlarged due to excessive stimulation by abnormal circulatory immunoglobulins and where there is excess production of thyroid hormone by hyperactive thyroid nodules.

In young people the classic features of weight loss, hyperactivity, tremor, heat intolerance and sweating are too well known to need elaborating. In the elderly, cardiac dysrhythmias and failure may be the sole features, and diagnosis may be missed. Diagnosis is clinical, confirmed by a high serum T_4, with or without a high T_3 and a low TSH level.

The forms of treatment vary. Antithyroid drugs are used and of these *carbimazole* (Neo-mercazole$_{GB}$) or *methimazole* (Tapazole$_{US}$) is most commonly used commencing with 30 mg/day reducing to a maintenance dose of 5–15 mg/day and continuing for 12–18 months. Immediate control of symptoms alone can be achieved by the use of β-adrenergic blockers such as *propranolol* (Inderal$_{GB.US}$). When drug treatment fails in the under-45s (child-bearing age), partial thyroidectomy is the treatment of choice. Over 45 years with failed drug treatment, radio-iodine (^{131}I) is given for permanent suppression of the gland.

Dental significance

Apart from occasional tremor of the tongue and increased muscle tone, there are no oral manifestations of hyperthyroidism and no contraindications to routine dentistry, but general anaesthetics should be avoided and, if essential, administered in hospital.

Hypothyroidism

This may result from primary failure of the gland or be secondary to hypothalamic or pituitary disease. Primary failure may be due to idiopathic atrophy, deficient thyroid hormone synthesis, autoimmune disease (Hashimoto's), thyroiditis, surgical removal, malignant infiltration or irradiation (^{131}I). Though very familiar, the clinical features are often overlooked. The gross features, gruff voice, slowness of movement and expression, and puffy sallow features are obvious. Other, frequently missed, features include anaemia, mental changes and psychoses, alopecia, dry skin, menorrhagia, ataxia, polyneuritis and carpal tunnel syndrome. Diagnosis is confirmed by a low serum T_4 and high TSH levels in primary hypothyroidism. *L-Thyroxine sodium* (Eltroxin$_{GB}$, Choloxin$_{GB.US}$, Synthroid$_{US}$) is given (100–200 mg/day) taking particular care in the elderly who may develop cardiac complications and thus should be started on a smaller dose (50 mg/day) initially.

Certain special problems arise in hypothyroidism. Myxoedema coma is rare but often fatal. Neonatal hypothyroidism must be diagnosed early to prevent mental damage.

Dental significance

In long-standing hypothyroidism swelling of the tongue is common and, in the young, this is accompanied by anterior open bite and delayed eruption of teeth.

Hashimoto's disease (lymphadenoid goitre)

This is an autoimmune thyroid disease in which antibodies are formed to thyroglobulin and thyroid cells. Chronic inflammation occurs with gradual destruction of the gland. Hypothryoidism results and, if untreated, may proceed to myxoedema. Treatment is with daily *thyroxine* for life.

Dental significance

Provided the patients are euthyroid there are no contraindications to dental treatment and anaesthesia.

Goitre

Enlargement of the thyroid gland (goitre) may result from hyperthyroidism, or rarely carcinoma, but most commonly as a compensatory response to decrease in circulating thyroid hormone. Decreased thyroid hormone production may result from iodine lack, enzyme defects, antithyroid drugs, and autoimmune or other forms of thyroiditis. Most goitres do not require surgery, the best treatment being reassurance. *Thyroxine* should be tried but significant reduction in gland size is rarely achieved.

Dental significance

There is no dental significance.

THYROTOXICOSIS

For thyrotoxicosis, *see* Thyroid disease *above*.

TIC DOLOREUX

For tic doloreux, *see* Trigeminal neuralgia.

TINEA

The condition is caused by a fungus, the common sites of infection being:

1. The scalp (ringworm), where it is seen in children as a circular patch from which the hair has fallen out.
2. The groin (dhobie itch), where it presents as a red raised butterfly rash which is irritant.
3. The feet (athlete's foot), where it appears as vesicles and macerated skin between the toes.

The condition is more common in hot weather and frequently picked up in changing-rooms and from infected towels.

Treatment is with topical ointments containing *clotrimazole* (Canestan$_{GB}$, Mycelex$_{US}$) or *undecenoates* (Mycota$_{GB}$, Tineafax$_{GB}$) for most infections, but systemic treatment with *griseofulvin* (Fulcin$_{GB}$, Grisovin$_{GB}$, Fulvicin$_{US}$) 125 mg four times daily, will be required if the nails are infected.

Dental significance

There is no dental significance.

TONSILLITIS

This common disease, characterized by severe sore throat and marked general malaise, occurs predominantly in children and adolescents. The usual organism is a haemolytic streptococcus. The tonsils are swollen and inflamed with pus exuding from the crypts. Complications include peritonsillar abscess and acute suppurative otitis media.

Symptomatic treatment and *aspirin* or *paracetamol* are usually all that is required. Antibiotics, of which *penicillin V* 250 mg four times daily is the best to start with, should be reserved for follicular tonsillitis and tonsillar abscess (quinsy). A throat swab should be taken and sent for culture and sensitivity assessment.

It should be remembered that tonsillitis is an early feature of many infectious fevers. Tonsillectomy is considered for patients who suffer recurrent attacks of tonsillitis or otitis media.

Dental significance

Dental treatment should be postponed until the condition has subsided.

TOXOPLASMOSIS

The condition is caused by the parasite, *Toxoplasma gondii*, which can be transmitted to man as mature oocytes present in cat faeces, or through goat's milk or uncooked goat meat.

Most infections are subclinical and antibody tests are positive for 30% of the population in the UK. Transplacental spread occurs in a third of infected mothers with 30% of fetuses showing congenital defects.

The commonest presentation is simple lymphadenopathy, but in a number of cases other organs are involved or there may be generalized toxoplasmosis with a maculopapular rash and hepatosplenomegaly. Treatment is with *spiramycin* 2 g daily for 2 weeks, or *triple sulphonamide* or *pyrimethamine*.

Dental significance

Although rare, the condition should be borne in mind as a cause of symptomless cervical adenopathy, particularly in those closely associated with cats or goats.

Transmission of the infection via the dental surgery is unlikely.

TRACHEITIS

Acute tracheitis, together with laryngitis and bronchitis, is frequently the complication of a severe cold or influenza. The symptoms are well known. Although initially caused by a virus, secondary bacterial infection may follow.

Smoking should be avoided and bedrest and staying indoors is advisable. Inhalations three times a day and at night with compound benzoin tincture (5 ml in 500 ml hot water) is helpful, with a cough linctus and analgesics as required.

In the very young, the old, the infirm and those on immunosuppressive or cytotoxic drugs, antibiotic treatment should be given. *Ampicillin* 250 mg 6-hourly for adults and 12.5 mg/kg 6-hourly for children is probably the best, except for those sensitive to it.

Dental significance

Patients without severe dental discomfort should be advised to postpone treatment until recovered.

TRANSIENT ISCHAEMIC ATTACKS (TIAs)

By definition, these give rise to neurological symptoms lasting less than 24 hours. They are probably due in most cases to atherothromboembolism arising from disease in the carotid artery, but emboli arising from the heart are a frequent cause. The neurological deficit associated with migraine is considered a separate entity from TIAs. Although attacks are short lasting, approximately 5% per annum progress to a stroke.

Treatment is avoidance of risk factors, stopping smoking and control of hypertension. Aspirin may be helpful and recent research has indicated that its value is enhanced if given in combination with *dipyridamole* ($\text{Persantin}_{GB,US}$). In certain situations anticoagulation or surgery are indicated.

Dental significance

There is no dental significance.

TRANSPLANTATION

The development in techniques for matching donors to recipients, in surgical techniques, and in the management and prevention of rejection, has lead to an explosion in organ transplantation in recent years.

Patient survival after renal transplantation has risen to 95% at the end of the first year. Cardiac transplantation is now established in the management of certain types of end-stage disease, over 400 patients having undergone transplantation worldwide. Marrow transplantation has been performed with increasing frequency in the last 10 years for haematological malignancy and aplastic anaemia. Forty-five to fifty per cent of patients with aplastic anaemia are apparently cured compared with 10% for leukaemias. Liver, heart–lung and liver–heart–lung transplantations are being carried out with increasing frequency. Although still rare events nationwide, with increasing survival rates dental practitioners are increasingly likely to encounter such patients. Drugs given to avert rejection include *azathioprine* ($\text{Imuram}_{GB,US}$), *cyclosporin A* (Sandimmun_{GB}) and *prednisolone*.

Dental significance

Patients awaiting transplants should be rendered dentally fit and have a high standard of oral hygiene. After transplant surgery, operative dental surgery and deep scaling should only be undertaken with antibiotic cover, as for Heart disease, infective (*see* Infective endocarditis).

Cyclosporin is known to cause gingival hyperplasia, similar to that caused by *phenytoin* especially when prescribed in doses of 500 mg daily or over. Patients who are receiving *prednisolone*, or have been treated with it recently, need special precautions (*see* Addison's disease *under* Adrenal diseases).

TRIGEMINAL NEURALGIA

The cause of this distressing complaint remains unknown. It is more common in older women and is usually unilateral. The pain, which is severe, occurs in spasms lasting a few seconds to a minute, is precipitated by movement of the mouth or touching the face, and is felt over the distribution area of the maxillary or mandibular division of the trigeminal nerve. Occasionally the condition is associated with multiple sclerosis.

At the present time, *carbamazepine* ($\text{Tegretol}_{\text{GB, US}}$) is the treatment of choice, starting with a dose of 50 mg three times daily and increasing until the symptoms disappear or unpleasant side-effects such as dizziness or skin rashes occur (usually 200 mg three times daily). *Baclofen* ($\text{Lioresal}_{\text{GB, US}}$) has been used with success in a number of cases where the patient was unable to tolerate *carbamazepine*. Various surgical procedures, which include destruction or division of the nerve or ganglion, are available for those who are not helped by drug therapy, but their disadvantages need carefully explaining before they are undertaken. Peripheral cryotherapy and high frequency thermocoagulation of the ganglion are among the methods in modern use, but more recently vascular surgery to a loop of the cerebellar artery pressing on the nerve root has claimed a high success rate without unpleasant sequelae.

Dental significance

As the trigger point may be in or around the mouth and spasm provoked by cleaning the teeth, bad oral hygiene is not uncommon and patients may be very reluctant to submit to dental examination.

Intermittent attacks of acute pulpitis or pain from a damaged inferior dental nerve may cause similar symptoms, and must be considered in the differential diagnosis.

TUBERCULOSIS

Although much less common than it used to be, tuberculosis is still seen widely in this country, causing significant morbidity and mortality. Any system in the body can be involved so presentation may be extremely variable and diagnosis often very difficult. Two strains of *Mycobacterium tuberculosis*, human and bovine, cause disease in man.

Infection may be localized to the skin, lungs, gastrointestinal tract, kidneys, bones, lymph glands, liver, adrenals, meninges or joints, and symptoms are those of the involved system. When infected material enters the circulation, generalized disease results leading to miliary tuberculosis. This occurs in people with chronic tuberculosis or in the immunosuppressed. Symptoms become generalized and include fatigue, headache, weight loss, night sweats and fever.

The diagnosis is suspected by characteristic radiological or clinical findings and confirmed by demonstrating the bacillus in tissue or body secretions and growing it in culture or in guinea-pigs. The disadvantage of the latter method is the delay of 4 or more weeks waiting for the result.

The incidence of tuberculosis has been greatly reduced by the introduction of the BCG vaccine (bacillus of Calmette–Guérin), an attenuated strain of the tubercle bacillus. The Mantoux or Heaf skin test is used to assess immune status and, if negative, the vaccine is given. Vaccine should be offered to children from 10 to 13 years and to all immigrants.

The prognosis of tuberculosis has been radically altered by the refinement of antituberculous antibiotics. Treatment has two phases: an initial phase when at least three drugs are used for 8 weeks or more, and a continuation phase when the drugs are reduced to two for 9 months. Drugs of choice are *isoniazid* (up to 300 mg daily), *rifampicin* 450–600 mg daily, and *ethambutol* (Mynah$_{GB}$, Myambutol$_{GB, US}$) 15 mg/kg daily.

Dental significance

Tuberculous ulcers occur in the mouth, more commonly on the tongue, and are usually secondary to pulmonary infection. They have a ragged outline and are generally painful. The bacilli are too scanty to be identified from a smear, and biopsy and culture are required. Patients with suspected tuberculous ulcers should be referred to their doctor for general assessment.

Tuberculous infection of the cervical lymph glands is now less common. Initially the swollen gland is painful and discrete but later becomes bound to the skin and may discharge through a sinus.

Tuberculosis of the salivary glands, and tuberculous osteomyelitis of the mandible, are fortunately rare.

Early diagnosis and treatment are important components in the fight against TB and dentists should remain alert to signs of the disease in the head and neck, especially among recent immigrants.

TUBEROUS SCLEROSIS (EPILOIA)

This is a neurocutaneous disorder inherited as an autosomal dominant trait and characterized by facial naevi (adenoma sebaceum), epilepsy and mental retardation.

Dental significance

The hyperplasia of the sebaceous glands (adenoma sebaceum) frequently affects the lower lip.

TYPHOID (ENTERIC FEVER)

Typhoid results from infection by *Salmonella typhi*, a Gram-negative rod, and occurs in areas of poor hygiene or where food or drinking water has become contaminated by human sewage. It is primarily a bacteraemic illness with abdominal symptoms occurring at some stage. The organism is swallowed and crosses the gut to multiply in the mesenteric glands before disseminating. The incubation period is 10–14 days. The severity of the illness varies and may be no more than a mild transitory illness. However, classically, during the first week the symptoms are of malaise, lethargy, headache, fever and anorexia. The characteristic rose spots, 2–4 mm in diameter, occur in only 10–20% of cases. During the second week there is a persistent pyrexia, tachycardia, delirium, distended abdomen, diarrhoea and splenomegaly. During the third week, the temperature usually settles but in a small proportion the disease progresses with severe toxicity, coma and occasionally bowel perforation or haemorrhage. For many years, *chloramphenicol* was the treatment of choice; however, some strains are now resistant. *Amoxycillin* is as effective and an alternative to *chloramphenicol*. It is less toxic but more expensive. Whichever antibiotic is used, treatment should be for not less than 2 weeks.

Active immunization with two injections of vaccine (TAB) 4 weeks apart, or monovalent typhoid vaccine, is an essential part of preventative treatment.

Dental significance

Parotitis is an unpleasant complication of the disease and the dentist should be ready to advise on oral hygiene to help to avoid this.

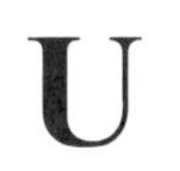

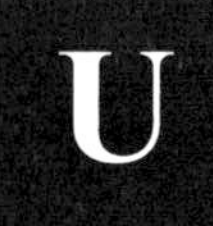

ULCERATIVE COLITIS

For ulcerative colitis, *see under* Colitis.

UNDULANT FEVER

For undulant fever, *see* Brucellosis.

URAEMIA

For uraemia, *see* Renal disease.

VARICELLA (CHICKEN POX)

Although more common in childhood, adults may catch the infection, when it tends to be more severe. The causative virus is the same as that of herpes zoster, and children may pick up chickenpox from an adult with shingles, but not the other way round.

The usual incubation period is 15–18 days and the condition frequently starts with general malaise and a prodromal erythematous rash. The characteristic vesicles appear first on the head and trunk and spread outwards.

As yet there is no vaccine against varicella and treatment is symptomatic with mild analgesics and *lotio calamine* and/or *trimeprazine* (Vallergan$_{GB}$, Temaril$_{US}$) to reduce the irriation. With immunodeficiency, the infection may be severe and intravenous *acyclovir* (Zovirax$_{GB,US}$) is proving helpful.

Dental significance

Vesicles may occur in the mouth, more commonly on the palate or fauces. They quickly break down to small ulcers with a surrounding area of erythema, which cause little discomfort and no treatment is required.

Dentists should appreciate the infectivity of the condition particularly in the early stages and/or with lesions in the mouth, and prevent suspected cases coming in contact with other children. After examination, instruments and the rinse-out glass should be thoroughly sterilized.

VASCULAR DISEASE

Arterial aneurysm

An aneurysm is a permanent dilatation of an artery due to destruction of its wall. It may be congenital, traumatic, inflammatory or degenerative.

Congenital aneurysms are confined to the base of the brain in the circle of Willis. The so-called 'Berry' aneurysm results from a defect of the media. Rupture leads to subarachnoid haemorrhage (*see under* Intracranial haemorrhage).

Traumatic aneurysms result from penetrating injuries such as gunshot wounds.

Inflammation due to such diseases as syphilis, bacterial endocarditis, and polyarteritis nodosum may cause aneurysms. Syphilis affects the aorta. Mycotic aneurysms result from infected emboli and are seen in infective endocarditis.

Atheroma is the commonest degenerative lesion causing aneurysm formation. The aorta may be affected at any site but most commonly in the abdomen below the renal arteries. Pain or awareness of abdominal pulsation are the most frequent symptoms although commonly no symptoms precede aneurysmal rupture. An aneurysm may be a chance finding on examination. Complications include rupture, thrombosis and embolism. Treatment when possible is surgical.

Dental significance

This is as for atheroma.

Atheroma

This is the commonest form of arterial degeneration. It is a generalized disease increasing with age, affecting particularly the arteries of the heart, brain, kidneys and limbs. Arterial narrowing results from a combination of atheromatous plaque formation and internal thrombosis. It may result in progressive impairment of blood supply. In the coronary arteries this causes angina and infarction, in the kidneys renal failure, in the cerebral arteries dementia and cerebrovascular accidents, and in the legs claudication, ischaemia and gangrene.

The cause of atheroma is obscure but high cholesterol level, high intake of saturated animal fats, hypertension and diabetes are all important factors in its development.

Dental significance

Because of their abundant blood supply, structures of the mouth are seldom affected by atheroma, although it may be found in the arteries supplying them.

Sometimes the pain of angina pectoris may be referred to the mouth or throat and suggests an oral pathology.

Patients with atheroma can be offered the full scope of dental treatment, but aspirating syringes and local anaesthetic without *adrenaline* should always be used and haemostatic string or packs containing *adrenaline* avoided. The hazard of general anaesthetics is increased in patients with the condition, but it can be justifiably claimed that, in a nervous patient, the anxiety of a dental extraction with local anaesthesia can be equally damaging. Providing the atheromatous condition is not advanced, short general anaesthetics can be given in the surgery making sure that anaesthetic gases always contain 50% oxygen.

Stroke

Cerebral thrombosis, haemorrhage and embolism lead to brain damage and infarction of the area of the brain supplied by the occluded vessel or damaged by the haemorrhage. The resulting neurological deficit, which may vary from minimal impairment of function to gross paralysis, is termed a 'stroke' or 'cerebrovascular accident'.

Cerebral atheroma and hypertension are major factors underlying strokes. Thromboses are commoner than haemorrhages, which are more often rapidly fatal. The commonest site for both is in the territory of the middle cerebral artery in the internal capsule.

In the carotid system the most common feature is a hemiplegia often accompanied by visual impairment and, if in the dominant hemispere, impairment of speech as well. The vertebral system, when involved, may give rise to a mixture of signs. Damage to long tracts causes hemiplegia, but in addition damage to brain stem, cranial nerve nuclei and their tracts results in a variety of cranial nerve defects and damage to cerebellar pathways causing ataxia.

Management is aimed at carefully graded rehabilitation with close cooperation between doctor, physiotherapist, occupational therapist and nurse. There is little place for anticoagulants. Hypertension should be treated but not too precipitously.

Occasionally the neurological signs of a stroke are fleeting and disappear. Such an event is termed a 'transient ischaemic attack' (TIA). In the majority of patients with such attacks a definitive stroke usually occurs within a year. It is therefore important to consider further investigations in this group in an attempt to find treatable lesions and prevent further strokes occurring. These patients may be helped by low-dose *aspirin* 300 mg daily.

Dental significance

Advice and assistance with oral hygiene is important if paralysis involves structures of the mouth. Conservation of the natural dentition is advisable as these patients frequently have trouble managing dentures. It is wise to use local anaesthetics without *adrenaline* and administer general anaesthetics in hospital.

VERTEBROBASILAR INSUFFICIENCY

Interference of blood flow through the vertebral arteries or basilar artery either due to atheromatous disease or external compression in the vertebral foramina may lead to dizzy turns and collapse with transient loss of consciousness. When this is due to degenerative changes in the cervical spine, attacks may be precipitated by neck movements, especially upward gaze. The wearing of a soft collar may limit neck movements and reduce attacks.

Dental significance

Extension of the neck in the dental chair should be guarded against, and general anaesthetics avoided.

VITAMIN DEFICIENCIES

Vitamin A (retinol)

Vitamin A is present in green vegetables, milk, and animal fats. Deficiency, which is seldom seen in the UK, causes xerophthalmia, conjunctival ulceration and night-blindness.

Dental significance

Xerostomia and keratinization in the mouth have been observed in vitamin A deficiency.

Vitamin B_1 (thiamine)

Deficiency causes beri-beri, a disease uncommon in the UK but sometimes seen in alcoholics. Symptoms include polyneuritis, muscle weakness, encephalopathy (Wernicke's encephalopathy) and cardiac failure. A sore mouth and secondary candida infection may be found on occasions.

Vitamin B_2 (riboflavin)

Deficiency results in changes in the skin and mucous membranes. Seborrhoeic dermatitis, a bright red tongue, and angular cheilitis are the common symptoms. Vascularization of the cornea occurs and is a diagnostic point. Treatment by taking brewers' yeast or vitamin B_2 10 mg daily corrects the deficiency.

Vitamin B_6 (pyridoxine)

Deficiency is rare but has been reported in patients with tuberculosis being treated with *isoniazid*. Muscle weakness, neuritis and stomatoglossitis are the common symptoms. Deficiency should be corrected by taking pyridoxine 30–60 mg daily.

Nicotinic acid

Deficiency, not normally seen in the UK, causes pellagra, whose features include dermatitis, erythema of the mucosa with papillary atrophy of the tongue, together with neurological disorders.

Vitamin B_{12}

The daily requirement of this vitamin, found only in animal products, is very small indeed and signs of deficiency usually result from a failure to absorb it. The clinical picture and oral manifestations are described under Anaemia.

Folic acid

Folic acid is present in yeast, green vegetables and animal products. The body requirements are small but deficiency can occur in pregnant women, alcoholics, the old and the debilitated. Certain lesions of the alimentary tract such as coeliac and Crohn's diseases can interfere with its absorption, and various drugs act as antagonists, notably *methotrexate* (a cytotoxic drug), *trimethoprim* (an antibacterial) and most anticonvulsant drugs (*phenobarbitone* and *phenytoin*).

The clinical picture produced by folic acid deficiency is identical to that of pernicious anaemia except for the neurological features which complicate vitamin B_{12} deficency (*see* Subacute combined degeneration of the cord), and the differential diagnosis can only be made by microbiological and radioassay tests.

Oral administration of folic acid in a dosage of 5 mg three times daily corrects the deficiency but should be administered with care as it has a potential hazard of exacerbating subacute combined degeneration of the cord in undiagnosed vitamin B_{12} deficiency.

Dental significance

The deficiency should be borne in mind in the class of patients susceptible, when the dentist is presented with a 'raw beef' tongue, recurrent mouth ulcers and angular cheilitis.

Vitamin C (ascorbic acid)

Deficiency of vitamin C, the vitamin of citrus fruit and fresh vegetables, leads to scurvy with swelling and ulceration of the gums and bleeding at the gingival margin. The diagnosis is confirmed by assaying the leucocyte vitamin C concentration, a reading of less than 10 μg/10^6 cells being positive.

Overt clinical scurvy is now rare in the UK, but recent research has shown that up to 50% of the elderly and debilitated have leucocyte levels of vitamin C down to scurvy level in the winter months. Vitamin C is important in the synthesis of collagen, and as such plays a part in the healing of wounds; but other properties, such as stimulating leucocyte function and aiding immune responses, remain unproven.

Vitamin C, taken by mouth in a daily dosage of 100 mg, is sufficient to correct any deficiency. Higher dosage appears harmless but unnecessary.

Dental significance

Gingival inflammation of the elderly during the winter months should raise suspicions of vitamin C deficiency and, as vitamin C supplement is simple and harmless, it should be prescribed if no other pathology is obvious.

Vitamin D (cholecalciferol)

Deficiency of vitamin D causes rickets in the young and osteomalacia in adults. Its main dietary sources are eggs, butter, milk and fish-liver oils. It is also formed in the skin under the influence of sunlight. The symptoms of rickets are painful swellings at the ends of the long bones and ribs (rickety rosary), frontoparietal bosses on the skull and muscle weakness. Severe bone pain is a characteristic of osteomalacia, especially at the sites of pseudofractures (Looser's zone).

The condition is seen in the UK more commonly in Asian immigrants, the elderly and housebound, and those on treatment with anticonvulsants or *aluminium hydroxide*.

Renal rickets results from failure in renal metabolism of vitamin D.

Treatment is with vitamin D 2000 units daily in dietary insufficiency. For renal rickets and hypoparathyroidism very large doses (50 000–150 000 units per day) are required.

Dental significance

Surprisingly, the teeth are little affected and enamel hypoplasia is rare. X-rays may show elongation of the pulp horns and, in the mandible and maxilla, there is diminished thickness of cortical bone and the lamina dura. Dental abscesses may occur through the extended pulp horns being opened up to the mouth as a result of attrition.

Vitamin E

Except perhaps in premature infants, there is doubt about the necessity of this substance. No oral manifestations of deficiency have been recorded.

Vitamins K_1 and K_2

Vitamin K_1 is found in green vegetables and vitamin K_2 is synthesized by bacteria in the intestine. Together they are essential for the synthesis of various factors in clotting of the blood.

Deficiency usually results from either a sterile gut, as in the newborn, or from malabsorption as a result of obstructive jaundice or steatorrhoea, particularly in the face of oral antibiotic therapy. Anticoagulants act competitively with vitamin K and prevent the synthesis of clotting factors.

Where there is deficiency, vitamin K is best given by intramuscular injection (10–20 mg).

Dental significance

Patients with conditions which predispose to vitamin K deficiency are at risk with surgery or extractions, and should be given vitamin K supplement, *menadiol sodium phosphate* (Synkavit$_{GB, US}$), 6–8 hours prior to operation.

VON RECKLINGHAUSEN'S DISEASE

For von Recklinghausen's disease, *see* Neurofibromatosis.

VON WILLEBRAND'S DISEASE

For von Willebrand's disease, *see* Haemophilia, Christmas disease and von Willebrand's disease.

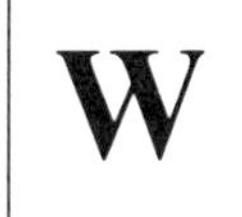

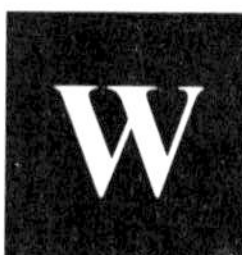

WALDENSTRÖM'S MACROGLOBULINAEMIA

For Waldenström's macroglobulinaemia, *see* Macroglobulinaemia.

WATERHOUSE–FRIDERICHSEN SYNDROME (FULMINATING MENINGOCOCCAL SEPTICAEMIA)

This is an overwhelming septicaemic illness associated with haemorrhages into the adrenal cortices and elsewhere, in which death is usual within 4–24 hours of onset. It most commonly occurs in young children. If the diagnosis can be made early enough, life can be saved.

Dental significance

There is no dental significance.

WEGENER'S GRANULOMA

This is probably a variant of polyarteritis nodosum, characterized by ulcerating nasal granulomata and necrotic lesions in the lung. It occurs in middle life, equally in both sexes, and is accompanied by fever, cough, haemoptysis and pleurisy. Prognosis is poor but may be improved by treatment with corticosteroids.

Dental significance

The condition also involves the mouth, where it takes the form of granulomatous swelling of the interdental papillae with destruction of the alveolus below. Extraction sockets display the same picture and fail to heal properly.

WEIL'S DISEASE

For Weil's disease, *see* Leptospirosis.

WERNICKE'S ENCEPHALOPATHY

For Wernicke's encephalopathy, *see* Vitamin deficiencies – Vitamin B_1.

WHIPPLE'S DISEASE

This rare disorder, predominantly of middle-aged men, is characterized by malabsorption, arthritis and lymphadenopathy. Diagnosis is made by jejunal biopsy demonstrating distortion of mucosal anatomy by large quantities of periodic acid–Schiff (PAS) material in the lamina propria. This is the end-product of bacterial degradation and a small rod-shaped organism has been demonstrated in the mucosa. The condition responds well to *tetracycline* 250 mg four times a day for 2 years.

Dental significance

There is no dental significance.

WHOOPING COUGH

For whooping cough, *see* Pertussis.

WILSON'S DISEASE

For Wilson's disease, *see under* Liver disease – Cirrhosis.

WOLFF–PARKINSON–WHITE SYNDROME

For Wolff–Parkinson–White syndrome, *see under* Heart disease, dysrhythmias – Paroxysmal atrial tachycardia.

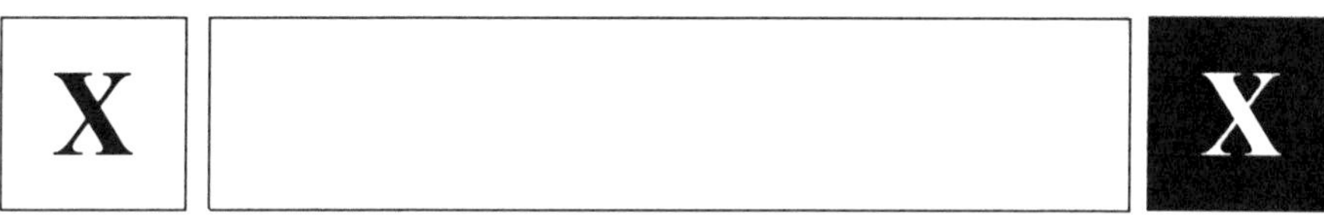

XANTHOMATOSES

For xanthomatoses, *see* Hyperlipidaemias.

Z

ZOLLINGER–ELLISON SYNDROME

The symptoms of this condition result from excessive gastric acid secretion due to non-B-cell adenoma or islet cell hyperplasia of the pancreas producing abnormal quantities of gastrin. Abnormal and extensive peptic ulceration occurs extending into the second part of the duodenum. Diarrhoea, bleeding and perforation are complications. Diagnosis is confirmed by grossly raised serum gastrin levels and treatment, where possible, is excision of the tumour and gastrectomy. Where surgery is not possible medical control with H_2-receptor antagonists, *cimetidine* (Tagamet$_{GB, US}$) or *ranitidine* (Zantac$_{GB}$) has been very successful.

Dental significance

This is as for peptic ulcer.

ZOSTER

For zoster, *see* Herpes zoster.

Section 2

Weights, measures and normal values

Length	1 inch = 2.54 cm	1 cm = 0.34 inch
	1 ft = 30.5 cm	1 m = 3 ft 3 inches
Weight	1 oz = 28.35 g	1 g = 0.04 oz
	1 lb = 0.45 kg	1 kg = 2.21 lb
Volume	1 fl. oz = 28.41 ml	1 ml = 0.036 fl. oz
	1 pt = 568 ml	1 litre = 1.76 pt

NORMAL BLOOD VALUES

Haemoglobin (Hb)	Men	13.5–18 g/dl
	Women	11.5–16.4 g/dl
Red blood cell count (RBC)		$4.5–6.0 \times 10^{12}/l$ (4.5–6.0 million per mm^3)
Mean corpuscular haemoglobin (MCH)		27–35 pg
Mean corpuscular volume (MCV)		76–96 fl (76–96 μm^3)
Packed cell volume (PCV)	Men	40–54%
	Women	36–47%
White blood cell count (WBC)		$4–10 \times 10^9/l$ (4000–10 000/mm^3)
Neutrophils		40–75%
Lymphocytes		20–50%
Monocytes		2–10%
Eosinophils		1–6%
Basophils		< 1%
Platelets		$150–400 \times 10^9/l$ (150 000–400 000/mm^3)
ESR		0–8 mm/h
Acid phosphatase		3.5–20 iu/l
Alkaline phosphatase		30–105 iu/l

Aspartate transaminase	7–35 iu/l
Bicarbonate	24–32 mmol/l
Bilirubin	1–17 mmol/l
Calcium	2.12–2.62 mmol/l
Chloride	95–105 mmol/l
Creatinine	64–124 mmol/l
Glucose	3.3–6.0 mmol/l
Lipids	
Cholesterol	3.6–6.5 mmol/l
Triglycerides	0.3–1.8 mmol/l
Potassium	3.5–5.0 mmol/l
Protein (total)	60–80 g/l
Albumin	35–50 g/l
Sodium	135–145 mmol/l
Urea	2.5–6.6 mmol/l
Uric acid	150–480 μmol/l
Bleeding time	< 9.5 minutes
Clotting time	10–12 minutes
International Normalized Ratio (INR) (prothrombin time)	0.9–1.1
Partial thromboplastin time (PTTK)	up to 50 seconds
Thrombin time	15–17 seconds

Section 3

Alphabetical list of pharmacological and proprietary drug names

acebutolol$_{GB,US}$	Sectral$_{GB,US}$, a β-blocker
Acepril$_{GB}$	*see captopril*$_{GB}$, angiotensin-converting enzyme (ACE) inhibitor used in treatment of hypertension and heart failure
acetaminophen$_{US}$	Tylenol$_{US}$, mild analgesic
acetazolamide$_{GB,US}$	Diamox$_{GB,US}$, carbonic anhydrase inhibitor, used in glaucoma
acetohexamide$_{GB,US}$	Dimelor$_{GB,US}$, hypoglycaemic agent
acetylcysteine$_{GB,US}$	Fabrol$_{GB}$, Mucomyst$_{GB,US}$, mucolytic Parvolex$_{GB}$, antidote for paracetamol poisoning
Achromycin$_{GB,US}$	*see tetracycline*
Actal$_{GB}$	*see alexitol sodium*$_{GB}$, antacid
Acthar$_{GB,US}$	*see corticotrophin*$_{GB,US}$
Actifed$_{GB,US}$	cough compound
actinomycin$_{GB}$	Cosmegen Lyovac$_{GB,US}$, cytotoxic antibiotic, main use in childhood solid tumours, causes marrow depression
Acupan$_{GB}$	*see nefopam*$_{GB}$
acyclovir$_{GB,US}$	Zovirax$_{GB,US}$, antiviral agent effective against herpes simplex and to lesser extent against herpes zoster
Adalat$_{GB,US}$	*see nifedipine*
Adcortyl$_{GB}$	*see triamcinolone*$_{GB,US}$
adrenocorticotrophic hormone$_{GB}$	*see corticotrophin*$_{GB}$
Albucid$_{GB}$	*see sulphacetamide*$_{GB,US}$
Aldactide$_{GB}$	*see spironolactone*$_{GB,US}$ and *hydroflumethiazide*$_{GB,US}$
Aldactone$_{GB,US}$	*see spironolactone*$_{GB,US}$
Aldomet$_{GB,US}$	*see methyldopa*$_{GB,US}$
alexitol sodium	Actal$_{GB}$, antacid
Alkeran$_{GB,US}$	*see melphalan*$_{GB,US}$
allopurinol$_{GB,US}$	Zyloric$_{GB}$, Lopurin$_{US}$, Zyloprim$_{US}$, xanthine oxidase inhibitor for treatment of hyperuricaemia
Altacite$_{GB}$	*see hydrotalcite*$_{GB}$
Aludrox$_{GB,US}$	*see aluminium hydroxide*$_{GB,US}$

amoxycillin$_{GB,US}$	Amoxil$_{GB,US}$, ampicillin derivative with similar antibacterial spectrum, but twice as well absorbed by mouth
amphetamine$_{GB,US}$	Benzedrine$_{US}$, central nervous stimulant, its use may lead to dependence and psychotic states
amphotericin$_{GB,US}$	Fungilin$_{GB}$, Mysteclin$_{US}$, antifungal drug which can be given systemically
ampicillin$_{GB,US}$	Penbritin$_{GB}$, Amcill$_{US}$, antibiotic active against certain Gram-positive and Gram-negative organisms, but inactivated by penicillinases, may affect the absorption of oral contraceptives
Ampiclox$_{GB}$	*ampicillin*$_{GB,US}$ + *cloxicillin*$_{GB,US}$
amylobarbitone$_{GB}$	a hypnotic and sedative – little used now
Amytal$_{GB,US}$	*see amylobarbitone*$_{GB}$
Anafranil$_{GB}$	*see clomipramine*$_{GB}$
Andursil$_{GB}$	antacid mixture
Antabuse$_{GB,US}$	*see disulfiram*
Antepar$_{GB,US}$	*see piperazine*$_{GB,US}$
aluminium hydroxide$_{GB,US}$	antacid, reduces absorption of tetracyclines
Alupent$_{GB,US}$	*see orciprenaline*$_{GB}$
amantadine$_{GB,US}$	Symmetrel$_{GB,US}$, dopaminergic drug used in parkinsonism and prophylaxis and treatment of influenza
Amcill$_{US}$	*see ampicillin*$_{GB,US}$
Amicar$_{US}$	*see aminocaproic acid*$_{GB,US}$
amiloride$_{GB,US}$	Moduretic$_{GB,US}$, potassium-sparing diuretic
aminocaproic acid$_{GB,US}$	Epsikapron$_{GB}$, Amicar$_{US}$, antifibrinolytic drugs used for haemorrhage after surgery
aminophylline$_{GB,US}$	xanthine derivative used in asthma
amiodarone$_{GB,US}$	Cordarone$_{GB,US}$, antidysrhythmic agent, used only when other agents fail
Amitid$_{US}$	*see amitriptyline*$_{GB,US}$
amitriptyline$_{GB,US}$	Elavil$_{GB,US}$, Lentizol$_{GB}$, Tryptizol$_{GB}$, tricyclic antidepressant, causes a dry mouth, use local anaesthetics without adrenaline
Amoxil$_{GB,US}$	*see amoxycillin*$_{GB,US}$
Antepsin$_{GB}$	*see sucralfate*$_{GB}$

Anturan$_{GB,US}$	*see sulphinpyrazone*$_{GB,US}$
Apresoline$_{GB,US}$	*see hydralazine*$_{GB,US}$
Aprinox$_{GB}$	*see bendrofluazide*$_{GB,US}$
aprotinin$_{GB}$	Trasylol$_{GB}$, a proteolytic enzyme inhibitor used in acute pancreatitis
Aralen$_{US}$	*see chloroquine*$_{GB,US}$
Artane$_{GB,US}$	*see benzhexol*$_{GB,US}$
Asacol$_{GB}$	*see mesalazine*$_{GB}$
Asilone$_{GB}$	antacid mixture
aspirin$_{GB,US}$	analgesic, potentiates action of warfarin and oral hypoglycaemics slightly, absorption impaired by antacids
astemizole$_{GB}$	Hismanal$_{GB}$, antihistamine
atenolol$_{GB,US}$	Tenormin$_{GB}$, β-blocker, hypotensive effect of general anaesthetics potentiated
Ativan$_{GB,US}$	*see lorazepam*$_{GB,US}$
Atromid$_{GB,US}$	*see clofibrate*$_{GB,US}$
atropine$_{GB,US}$	anticholinergic drug, not to be given to patients with glaucoma
Atrovent$_{GB}$	*see ipratropium bromide*$_{GB}$
Augmentin$_{GB,US}$	amoxycillin, plus clavulanic acid, active against penicillinase-producing bacteria resistant to amoxycillin alone
Aureocort$_{GB}$	compound skin preparation
Aureomycin$_{GB,US}$	*see chlortetracycline*$_{GB,US}$
Avloclor$_{GB}$	*see chloroquine*$_{GB,US}$
azapropazone$_{GB}$	Rheumox$_{GB}$, non-steroidal anti-inflammatory drug
azathioprine$_{GB,US}$	Imuran$_{GB,US}$, immunosuppressant agent, used to prevent transplant rejection, and in certain other conditions, such as collagen disorders and Crohn's disease, may cause marrow depression
Azulfidine$_{US}$	*see sulphasalazine*$_{GB,US}$
baclofen$_{GB,US}$	Lioresal$_{GB,US}$, muscle relaxant: used for muscle spasm in spastic conditions
Bactrim$_{GB,US}$	*see co-trimoxazole*$_{GB,US}$
Baxan$_{GB}$	*see cefadroxil*$_{GB,US}$
beclomethasone$_{GB,US}$	Becotide$_{GB}$, Vanceril$_{US}$, corticosteroid used in aerosol inhalation or insufflation form for bronchospasm; occasionally suppresses adrenals, may cause pharyngeal candidiasis

Beconase$_{GB,US}$	*see beclomethasone*$_{GB,US}$
Becotide$_{GB}$	*see beclomethasone*$_{GB,US}$
belladonna$_{GB,US}$	anticholinergic agent, may cause dry mouth
bendrofluazide$_{GB}$	thiazide diuretic
Benemid$_{GB,US}$	*see probenecid*$_{GB,US}$
Benoral$_{GB}$	*see benorylate*$_{GB}$
benorylate$_{GB}$	non-steroidal anti-inflammatory agent
benserazide$_{GB}$	(with levodopa in Madopar$_{GB}$) extracerebral dopa-decarboxylase inhibitor for parkinsonism
Benzedrine$_{US}$	*see amphetamine*$_{GB,US}$
benzhexol$_{GB}$	Artane$_{GB,US}$, anticholinergic drug used in parkinsonism, may cause a dry mouth
benzodiazepines	hypnotic, sedative and anxiolytic drugs
benzyl benzoate$_{GB}$	Ascabiol$_{GB}$, treatment of scabies
benzylpenicillin$_{GB}$	Crystapen$_{GB}$, antibiotic; also known as penicillin G
Berotec$_{GB}$	*see fenoterol hydrobromide*$_{GB}$
Beta-Cardone$_{GB}$	*see sotalol*$_{GB}$
Betadine$_{GB,US}$	*povidone–iodine*$_{GB,US}$, antiseptic
betahistine hydrochloride$_{GB}$	Serc$_{GB}$, for vertigo and hearing disturbances in labyrinthine disorders
Betaloc$_{GB}$	*see metoprolol*$_{GB,US}$
betamethasone$_{GB,US}$	corticosteroid with little mineralocorticoid action, useful in certain dermatological disorders, may suppress adrenals
bethanidine$_{GB}$	Esbatal$_{GB}$, adrenergic-neurone blocking hypotensive agent, can cause discomfort in salivary glands, potentiates hypotensive effect of general anaesthetics
Betim$_{GB}$	*see timolol maleate*$_{GB}$
Betnovate$_{GB}$	compound skin preparation
Bextasol$_{GB}$	*see betamethasone valerate*$_{GB,US}$
bezafibrate$_{GB}$	Bezalip$_{GB}$, used in treatment of hyperlipidaemia
Bezalip$_{GB}$	*see bezafibrate*$_{GB}$
Biogastrone$_{GB}$	*see carbenoxolone sodium*$_{GB}$
Bioplex$_{GB}$	*see carbenoxolone*$_{GB}$
bisacodyl$_{GB,US}$	Dulcolax$_{GB,US}$, powerful stimulant laxative
Blenoxane$_{US}$	*see bleomycin*$_{GB,US}$

bleomycin$_{GB,US}$	Blenoxane$_{US}$, cytotoxic agent, causes marrow suppression
Blocadren$_{GB,US}$	*see timolol*$_{GB,US}$
Bolvidon$_{GB}$	*see mianserin*$_{GB}$
Bonjela$_{GB}$	*see choline salicylate*$_{GB,US}$
Bricanyl$_{GB,US}$	*see terbutaline*$_{GB,US}$
bromocriptine$_{GB,US}$	Parlodel$_{GB,US}$, stimulates dopamine receptors used in parkinsonism
Brufen$_{GB,US}$	*see ibuprofen*$_{GB,US}$
bumetanide$_{GB,US}$	Burinex$_{GB}$, Bumax$_{US}$, loop diuretic
buprenorphine$_{GB,US}$	Temgesic$_{GB}$, Buprenex$_{US}$, powerful analgesic, not to be used in patients taking monoamine oxidase inhibitors
Burinex$_{GB}$	*see bumetanide*$_{GB}$
Buscopan$_{GB}$	*see hyoscine*$_{GB,US}$
busulphan$_{GB,US}$	Myleran$_{GB,US}$, cytotoxic agent, causes marrow depression
Butacote$_{GB}$	*see phenylbutazone*$_{GB,US}$
Butazolidin$_{GB,US}$	*see phenylbutazone*$_{GB,US}$
butobarbital$_{US}$	Soneryl$_{GB}$, barbiturate
butobarbitone$_{GB}$	Soneryl$_{GB}$, barbiturate
Cafergot$_{GB,US}$	*see ergotamine tartrate*
Caladryl$_{GB,US}$	compound skin preparation
calamine$_{GB,US}$	Caladryl$_{GB,US}$, local antipruritic agent
calciferol$_{GB,US}$	vitamin D
Calcimar$_{US}$	*see calcitonin*$_{GB,US}$
Calcitare$_{GB}$	*see calcitonin*$_{GB,US}$
calcitonin$_{GB,US}$	Calcitare$_{GB}$, Calcimar$_{US}$, lowers serum calcium level – used in Paget's disease and hyperparathyroidism
Canesten cream$_{GB}$	*see clotrimazole*$_{GB,US}$
Capoten$_{GB,US}$	*see captopril*$_{GB,US}$
captopril$_{GB,US}$	used in treatment of hypertensions; loss of taste and a scalding sensation in the mouth have been reported; general anaesthetics to be avoided
carbachol$_{GB}$	mydriatic
carbamazepine$_{GB,US}$	Tegretol$_{GB,US}$, anti-epileptic and used trigeminal neuralgia, reduces effect of oral contraceptives and anticoagulants and not to be given within 2 weeks of monoamine oxidase inhibitors
carbenicillin$_{GB,US}$	Pyopen$_{GB,US}$, antipseudomonal penicillin

carbenoxolone sodium$_{GB}$ — Biogastrone$_{GB}$, Duogastrone$_{GB}$ for peptic ulcer healing, also Bioplex$_{GB}$ for oral ulceration

carbidopa$_{GB,US}$ — Sinemet$_{GB,US}$, dopaminergic drug for parkinsonism, avoid use of halothane

carbimazole$_{GB}$ — antithyroid drug

Cardene$_{GB}$ — *see nicardipine*$_{GB}$

Catapres$_{GB,US}$ — *see clonidine*$_{GB,US}$

Caved-S$_{GB}$ — deglycyrrhizinized liquorice

CCNU$_{GB}$ — *see lomustine*$_{GB,US}$

cefaclor$_{GB,US}$ — Distaclor$_{GB}$, Ceclor$_{US}$, cephalosporin

cefadroxil$_{GB,US}$ — Baxan$_{GB}$, Duricef$_{US}$, a new oral cephalosporin

cefotaxime$_{GB,US}$ — Claforan$_{GB,US}$, a third generation cephalosporin

cefoxitin$_{GB,US}$ — Mefoxin$_{GB,US}$, cephalosporin antibiotic

cefuroxime$_{GB,US}$ — Zinacef$_{GB,US}$, cephalosporin antibiotic

Celevac$_{GB}$ — *see* methylcellulose$_{GB,US}$

cephalexin$_{GB,US}$ — Ceporex$_{GB}$, Keflex$_{GB,US}$, cephalosporin antibiotic

cephalothin$_{GB,US}$ — Keflin$_{GB,US}$, cephalosporin antibiotic

cephazolin$_{GB}$ — Kefzol$_{GB,US}$, cephalosporin antibiotic

cephradine$_{GB,US}$ — Velosef$_{GB,US}$, cephalosporin antibiotic

Ceporex$_{GB}$ — *see cephalexin*$_{GB,US}$

Cetiprin$_{GB}$ — *see emepronium bromide*$_{GB}$

chenodeoxycholic acid$_{GB}$ — Chendol$_{GB}$, Chenix$_{US}$, gallstone dissolving agent

chloral$_{GB,US}$ — hypnotic and sedative

chlorambucil$_{GB,US}$ — Leukeran$_{GB,US}$, alkylating cytotoxic drug causes marrow depression

chloramphenicol$_{GB,US}$ — Chloromycetin$_{GB,US}$, Kemicetine$_{GB}$, antibiotic, occasionally causes bone marrow depression

chlordiazepoxide$_{GB,US}$ — Librium$_{GB,US}$, anxiolytic agent

chlorhexidine$_{GB,US}$ — Corsodyl$_{GB}$, Peridex$_{US}$, oral antibacterial, as mouthwash or gel

chlormethiazole$_{GB}$ — Heminevrin$_{GB}$, hypnotic and sedative

Chloromycetin$_{GB,US}$ — *see chloramphenicol*$_{GB,US}$

chloroquine$_{GB,US}$ — Aralen$_{US}$, Avloclor$_{GB}$, antimalarial agent, can cause oral erosions

chlorothiazide$_{GB,US}$ — thiazide diuretic

chlorpheniramine$_{GB,US}$ — Piriton$_{GB}$, antihistamine

chlorpromazine$_{GB,US}$	Largactil$_{GB}$, antipsychotic drug, hypotensive effect of general anaesthetics potentiated
chlorpropamide$_{GB,US}$	Diabinese$_{GB,US}$, hypoglycaemic agent, potentiated by aspirin, can cause oral erosions
chlortetracycline$_{GB,US}$	antibiotic
chlorthalidone$_{GB,US}$	Hygroton$_{GB,US}$, diuretic
cholecalciferol$_{GB}$	vitamin D
Choledyl$_{GB,US}$	*see choline theophyllinate*$_{GB}$
cholestyramine$_{GB,US}$	Questran$_{GB,US}$, ion-exchange resin used in hyperlipidaemia and liver disease
choline salicylate$_{GB,US}$	Bonjela$_{GB}$, pain relief in mouth ulceration
choline theophyllinate$_{GB}$	Choledyl$_{GB}$, bronchodilator
cimetidine$_{GB,US}$	Tagamet$_{GB,US}$, H_2-receptor antagonist used for treatment of peptic ulcers, effect of diazepam is extended, absorption of tetracyclines reduced
cinnarizine$_{GB}$	Stugeron$_{GB}$, used for nausea and vomiting
ciprofloxacin$_{GB}$	Ciproxin$_{GB}$, a 4-quinolone antimicrobial with a wide spectrum, should not be used in conjunction with theophylline
Ciproxin$_{GB}$	*see ciprofloxacin*
cisplatin$_{GB,US}$	Neoplatin$_{GB}$, Platinol$_{US}$, alkylating agent used in the treatment of solid tumours
Claforan$_{GB}$	*see cefotaxime*$_{GB}$
Cleocin$_{US}$	*see clindamycin*$_{GB,US}$
clindamycin$_{GB,US}$	Dalacin C$_{GB}$, Cleocin$_{US}$, antibiotic, may cause pseudomembranous colitis
Clinoril$_{GB,US}$	*see sulindac*$_{GB,US}$
clobazam$_{GB}$	Frisium$_{GB}$, benzodiazepine anxiolytic
clobetasol proprionate$_{GB,US}$	Dermovate$_{GB}$, Temovate$_{US}$, topical steroid
clofibrate$_{GB,US}$	Atromid$_{GB,US}$, for hyperlipidaemia
clomiphene$_{GB,US}$	Clomid$_{GB,US}$, an anti-oestrogen for inducing ovulation
clomipramine$_{GB}$	Anafranil$_{GB}$, tricyclic antidepressant, use local anaesthetics without adrenaline
clonazepam$_{GB,US}$	Rivotril$_{GB}$, Clonopin$_{US}$, for epilepsy and myoclonic jerks
clonidine$_{GB,US}$	Catapres$_{GB,US}$, Dixarit$_{GB}$, hypotensive

	agent, may cause discomfort in salivary glands
Clonopin$_{US}$	*see clonazepam*$_{GB,US}$
clorazepate dipotassium$_{GB,US}$	Tranxene$_{GB,US}$, benzodiazepine anxiolytic agent
clotrimazole$_{GB,US}$	Canesten$_{GB}$, Mycelex$_{US}$, antifungal agent
cloxacillin$_{GB,US}$	Tegopen$_{US}$, antibiotic used for infections due to penicillinase-producing staphylococci
Co-betaloc$_{GB}$	*see metoprolol*$_{GB,US}$
co-dergocrine mesylate$_{GB}$	Hydergine$_{GB,US}$, cerebral vasodilator
cocaine$_{GB,US}$	an addictive drug causing central nervous stimulation
codeine phosphate$_{GB,US}$	analgesic, antidiarrhoeal agent
Codis$_{GB}$	*aspirin*$_{GB,US}$ and *codeine phosphate*$_{GB,US}$
colchicine$_{GB,US}$	used in acute gout
Colifoam$_{GB}$	steroid enema in foam form, used in colitis
colistin$_{GB,US}$	a polymyxin antibiotic used against Gram-negative organisms
Colofac$_{GB}$	*see mebeverine*$_{GB}$
Colpermin$_{GB}$	peppermint preparation for the relief of abdominal colic
Colven$_{GB}$	combined antispasmodic bulking agent for irritable bowel syndrome
Compazine$_{US}$	*see prochlorperazine*$_{GB,US}$
Concordin$_{GB}$	*see proptriptyline*$_{GB,US}$
Co-proxamol$_{GB}$	compound analgesic, paracetamol and dextropropoxyphene
Cordarone$_{GB}$	*see amiodarone*$_{GB}$
Cordilox$_{GB}$	*see verapamil*$_{GB}$
Corgard$_{GB,US}$	*see nadolol*$_{GB,US}$
Corsodyl$_{GB}$	*see chlorhexidine*$_{GB,US}$
corticotrophin$_{GB}$	Acthar$_{GB}$, used as alternative to cortisone and does not suppress adrenals
cortisone acetate$_{GB,US}$	a corticosteroid, causes adrenal suppression
Cotazym$_{GB,US}$	pancreatic supplement
co-trimoxazole$_{GB,US}$	Bactrim$_{GB,US}$, Septrin$_{GB}$, a mixture of sulphamethoxazole and trimethoprim, can enhance action of hypoglycaemics
Creon$_{GB}$	pancreatic enzyme preparation

Crystapen$_{GB}$	*benzylpenicillin*$_{GB}$
cromolyn sodium$_{US}$	Intal$_{GB,US}$, prophylactic agent in asthma
cyanocobalamin$_{GB,US}$	vitamin B_{12} preparation now largely replaced by hydroxocobalamin
cyclizine$_{GB,US}$	for nausea, vomiting and vertigo
cyclobarbitone$_{GB}$	barbiturate for severe intractable insomnia
cyclopenthiazide$_{GB}$	Navidrex$_{GB}$, diuretic
cyclophosphamide$_{GB,US}$	Endoxana$_{GB}$, Cytoxan$_{US}$, cytotoxic agent, causes marrow depression
cycloserine$_{GB,US}$	second line antituberculous agent
cyclosporin$_{GB,US}$	Sandimmun$_{GB,US}$, immunosuppressant, used in transplants; interacts with systemic antibiotics and ketoconazole, can cause gingival hypertrophy
Cyklokapron$_{GB}$	*see tranexamic acid*$_{GB}$
cyproheptadine$_{GB,US}$	Periactin$_{GB,US}$, antihistamine serotonin antagonist, used to stimulate appetite
Cytamen$_{GB}$	*see hydroxocobalamin*$_{GB}$
cytarabine$_{GB,US}$	Cytosar$_{US}$, cytotoxic agent, causes marrow depression
Cytosar$_{US}$	*see cytarabine*$_{GB,US}$
Cytoxan$_{US}$	*see cyclophosphamide*$_{GB,US}$

Daktarin$_{GB}$	*see miconazole*$_{GB,US}$
Dalacin$_{GB}$	*see clindamycin*$_{GB,US}$
Dalmane$_{GB,US}$	*see flurazepam*$_{GB,US}$
danazol$_{GB,US}$	Danol$_{GB}$, Danocrine$_{US}$, inhibitor of pituitary gonadotrophin secretion, used in treatment of endometriosis
Daonil$_{GB}$	*see glibenclamide*$_{GB}$
dapsone$_{GB,US}$	a sulphone antileprosy drug, may cause oral erosions
Daraprim$_{GB,US}$	*see pyrimethamine*$_{GB,US}$
DDAVP$_{GB}$	a vasopressin analogue for use in diabetes insipidus
debrisoquine sulphate$_{GB}$	Declinax$_{GB}$, adrenergic neurone-blocking drug for moderate to severe hypertension; hypotensive effect of general anaesthetics potentiated
Decadron$_{GB,US}$	*see dexamethasone*$_{GB,US}$
Declinax$_{GB}$	*see debrisoquine sulphate*
Declomycin$_{US}$	*see demeclocycline hydrochloride*$_{GB,US}$

deglycyrrhizinized liquorice$_{\mathrm{GB}}$	Caved-S$_{\mathrm{GB}}$, for treatment of peptic ulceration
demeclocycline hydrochloride$_{\mathrm{GB,US}}$	Ledermycin$_{\mathrm{GB}}$, Declomycin$_{\mathrm{US}}$, antibiotic
De-Nol$_{\mathrm{GB}}$	*see tripotassium dicitratobismuthate*$_{\mathrm{GB}}$
Depixol$_{\mathrm{GB}}$	*see flupenthixol*
Depo-Medrone$_{\mathrm{GB}}$	*see methylprednisolone*$_{\mathrm{GB,US}}$
Dermovate$_{\mathrm{GB}}$	*see clobetasol proprionate*$_{\mathrm{GB}}$
Deseril$_{\mathrm{GB}}$	*see methysergide*$_{\mathrm{GB,US}}$
desferrioxamine$_{\mathrm{GB,US}}$	Desferal$_{\mathrm{GB,US}}$, iron-chelating agent used for iron overload
Deteclo$_{\mathrm{GB}}$	*see tetracycline*$_{\mathrm{GB,US}}$
dexamethasone$_{\mathrm{GB,US}}$	Decadron$_{\mathrm{GB,US}}$, high-potency glucocorticoid with minimal mineralocorticoid action, may suppress adrenals
dexamphetamine$_{\mathrm{GB,US}}$	Dexedrine$_{\mathrm{GB,US}}$, central nervous system stimulant, may give rise to drug dependence
dextromoramide$_{\mathrm{GB}}$	Palfium$_{\mathrm{GB}}$, narcotic analgesic for severe pain; may lead to dependence; avoid in patients on monoamine oxidase inhibitors
dextropropoxyphene$_{\mathrm{GB}}$	Depronal$_{\mathrm{GB}}$, Distalgesic$_{\mathrm{GB}}$, narcotic analgesic for mild to moderate pain, potentiates carbamazepine
DF118$_{\mathrm{GB}}$	*see dihydrocodeine*$_{\mathrm{GB,US}}$
Diabinese$_{\mathrm{GB,US}}$	*see chlorpropamide*$_{\mathrm{GB,US}}$
diamorphine$_{\mathrm{GB}}$	*heroin*$_{\mathrm{GB}}$, powerful opiate analgesic likely to lead to dependence: not to be given to patients taking monoamine oxidase inhibitors
Diamox$_{\mathrm{GB,US}}$	*see acetazolamide*$_{\mathrm{GB,US}}$
diazepam$_{\mathrm{GB,US}}$	Valium$_{\mathrm{GB,US}}$, benzodiazepine hypnotic with a wide range of actions including anxiolytic premedication and anti-epileptic; effect prolonged by cimetidine; absorption delayed by antacids
diazoxide$_{\mathrm{GB,US}}$	Eudemine$_{\mathrm{GB}}$, vasodilator hypotensive, may cause hyperglycaemia
Dibenyline$_{\mathrm{GB}}$	*see phenoxybenzamine*$_{\mathrm{GB,US}}$
Dibenzyline$_{\mathrm{US}}$	*see phenoxybenzamine*$_{\mathrm{GB,US}}$

dichloralphenazone$_{\text{GB,US}}$	Welldorm$_{\text{GB,US}}$, mild sedative
diclofenac$_{\text{GB}}$	Voltarol$_{\text{GB}}$, non-steroidal anti-inflammatory agent
Diconal$_{\text{GB}}$	*see dipipanone*$_{\text{GB}}$
dicyclomine$_{\text{GB,US}}$	Merbentyl$_{\text{GB}}$, antispasmodic, may cause dry mouth
diethylpropion$_{\text{GB,US}}$	Apisate$_{\text{GB}}$, Tenuate$_{\text{GB,US}}$, centrally acting appetite suppressant
diflunisal$_{\text{GB,US}}$	Dolobid$_{\text{GB,US}}$, long-acting analgesic for mild to moderate pain
digoxin$_{\text{GB,US}}$	Lanoxin$_{\text{GB,US}}$, cardiac glycoside used in atrial dysrhythmias
dihydrocodeine$_{\text{GB,US}}$	DF118$_{\text{GB}}$, analgesic
Dilantin$_{\text{US}}$	*see phenytoin*$_{\text{GB,US}}$
diltiazem$_{\text{GB,US}}$	Tildiem$_{\text{GB}}$, Cardizem$_{\text{US}}$, calcium-channel blocker, used for angina
Dimelor$_{\text{GB}}$	*see acetohexamide*$_{\text{GB,US}}$
dimenhydrinate$_{\text{GB,US}}$	Dramamine$_{\text{GB,US}}$, antihistamine
Dindevan$_{\text{GB}}$	*see phenindione*$_{\text{GB}}$
Dioralyte	electrolyte powder or tablet reconstituted with water and used for oral fluid replacement
diphenhydramine$_{\text{GB,US}}$	Benadryl$_{\text{GB,US}}$, antihistamine
diphenoxylate$_{\text{GB,US}}$	Lomotil$_{\text{GB}}$, antidiarrhoeal agent, may cause a dry mouth
dipipanone$_{\text{GB}}$	Diconal$_{\text{GB}}$, opiate analgesic, not to be given to patients on monoamine oxidase inhibitors
dipyridamole$_{\text{GB,US}}$	Persantin$_{\text{GB,US}}$, antiplatelet agent
Disipal$_{\text{GB,US}}$	*see orphenadrine*$_{\text{GB,US}}$
disopyramide$_{\text{GB,US}}$	Rythmodan$_{\text{GB}}$, used in ventricular arrhythmias, may cause a dry mouth
Distaclor$_{\text{GB}}$	*see cefaclor*$_{\text{GB,US}}$
Distalgesic$_{\text{GB}}$	*see dextropropoxyphene*$_{\text{GB}}$
distigmine bromide$_{\text{GB}}$	Ubretid$_{\text{GB}}$, for urinary retention, interaction with halothane
disulfiram$_{\text{GB,US}}$	Antabuse$_{\text{GB,US}}$, used in the treatment of alcoholism, can cause acute psychosis with metronidazole
Dixarit$_{\text{GB}}$	*see clonidine*$_{\text{GB,US}}$
dobutamine$_{\text{GB}}$	Dobutrex$_{\text{GB}}$, inotropic support in hypertension; general anaesthetics should be given with caution
Dolobid$_{\text{GB}}$	*see diflunisal*$_{\text{GB}}$

domperidone$_{GB}$	Motilium$_{GB}$, used in nausea and vomiting
dopamine$_{GB,US}$	Intropin$_{GB,US}$, sympathomimetic agent used in cardiogenic shock
Doriden$_{GB,US}$	*see glutethimide*$_{GB,US}$
dothiepin$_{GB}$	Prothiaden$_{GB}$, tricyclic antidepressant, may cause a dry mouth, use local anaesthetics without adrenaline
doxapram$_{GB,US}$	a respiratory stimulant
doxorubicin hydrochloride$_{GB,US}$	cytotoxic agent
doxycycline$_{GB}$	Vibramycin$_{GB}$, a tetracycline antibiotic with a broad spectrum; stains teeth
Dramamine$_{GB,US}$	*see dimenhydrinate*$_{GB,US}$
droperidol$_{GB}$	Droleptan$_{GB}$, a tranquillizer for psychoses; avoid analgesics
Duogastrone$_{GB}$	*see carbenoxolone sodium*$_{GB}$
Duovent$_{GB}$	*fenoterol* and *ipratropium* in an aerosol
Duphalac$_{GB}$	*see lactulose*$_{GB}$
Duphaston$_{GB}$	*see dydrogesterone*$_{GB}$
Durabolin$_{GB,US}$	*see nandrolone*$_{GB,US}$
Dyazide$_{GB,US}$	*see triamterene*$_{GB,US}$
dydrogesterone$_{GB}$	Duphaston$_{GB}$, progestogen
Dytac$_{GB}$	*see triamterene*$_{GB,US}$
Dytide$_{GB}$	*see triamterene + benzthiazide*$_{GB,US}$
Edecrin$_{GB,US}$	*see ethacrynic acid*$_{GB,US}$
edrophonium$_{GB,US}$	used for diagnosis of myasthenia
Efcortelan$_{GB}$	hydrocortisone cream
Eltroxin$_{GB}$	*see thyroxine*$_{GB,US}$
emepronium bromide$_{GB}$	Cetiprin$_{GB}$, for urinary incontinence; oral and oesophageal ulceration have been described as complications
Emeside$_{GB}$	*see ethosuximide*$_{GB,US}$
emetine$_{GB}$	amoebicide
enalapril$_{GB,US}$	Innovace$_{GB}$, Vasotec$_{US}$, angiotensin-converting enzyme inhibitor, used in treatment of hypertension; hypotensive effect of general anaesthetics may be potentiated
Endoxana$_{GB}$	*see cyclophosphamide*$_{GB,US}$
Epanutin$_{GB}$	*see phenytoin*$_{GB,US}$
ephedrine$_{GB,US}$	for treatment of reversible airway obstruction
Epilim$_{GB}$	*see sodium valproate*$_{GB}$

Equagesic$_{GB,US}$	compound analgesic
Equanil$_{GB,US}$	*see meprobamate*$_{GB,US}$
ergotamine tartrate$_{GB,US}$	constricts arteries, used in migraine, potentiation by erythromycin has been reported
Erythrocin$_{GB,US}$	*see erythromycin*$_{GB,US}$
erythromycin$_{GB,US}$	Erythrocin$_{GB,US}$, Ilosone$_{GB,US}$, antibiotic with similar spectrum to penicillin and useful where there is penicillin allergy; Ilosone, which is erythromycin estolate, is better avoided in children
Esbatal$_{GB}$	*see bethanidine*$_{GB}$
ethacrynic acid$_{GB,US}$	Edecrin$_{GB,US}$, strong loop diuretic and of similar action to frusemide
ethambutol$_{GB,US}$	Mynah$_{GB}$, antituberculous drug; should be avoided in the very young and the elderly
ethionamide$_{GB,US}$	antituberculous drug used where resistance to first-line drugs occurs
ethosuximide$_{GB,US}$	Emeside$_{GB}$, Zarontin$_{GB,US}$, used in treatment of petit mal
Eugynon$_{GB}$	oral contraceptive, combined preparation
Fabrol$_{GB}$	*see acetylcysteine*$_{GB,US}$
famotidine$_{GB}$	Pepsid$_{GB}$, longer-acting H_2-receptor blocker for duodenal and gastric ulcers
Fansidar$_{GB,US}$	*see pyrimethamine*$_{GB,US}$ and *sulphadoxine*$_{GB,US}$
Fefol$_{GB}$	iron and folate preparation
Feldene$_{GB,US}$	*see piroxicam*$_{GB,US}$
fenbufen$_{GB}$	Lederfen$_{GB}$, non-steroidal anti-inflammatory; avoid aspirin
fenfluramine$_{GB,US}$	Ponderax$_{GB}$, Pondimim$_{US}$, appetite suppressant, may be a hazard for general anaesthetics
fenoprofen$_{GB,US}$	Progesic$_{GB}$, Nalfen$_{US}$, non-steroidal anti-inflammatory; avoid aspirin
fenoterol$_{GB}$	Berotec$_{GB}$, selective β_2-agonist used for treatment of asthma
Feospan$_{GB}$	*see ferrous sulphate* – a sustained release capsule
ferrous sulphate$_{GB,US}$	an oral iron preparation for treatment of iron deficiency anaemia

Flagyl$_{GB,US}$	*see metronidazole*$_{GB,US}$
flavoxate$_{GB,US}$	Urispas$_{GB,US}$, for urinary frequency and dysuria
flecainide$_{GB,US}$	Tambocor$_{GB,US}$, anti-arrhythmic agent for cardiac arrhythmias
Florinef$_{GB}$	*see fludrocortisone*$_{GB,US}$
Floxapen$_{GB}$	*see flucloxacillin*$_{GB}$
Fluanxol$_{GB}$	*see flupenthixol*$_{GB}$
flucloxacillin$_{GB}$	Floxapen$_{GB}$, penicillinase-resistant penicillin, for use in penicillin-resistant *Staphylococcus aureus* infections
fludrocortisone$_{GB,US}$	Florinef$_{GB}$, salt-retaining steroid used for replacement therapy in mineralocorticoid deficiency; may suppress adrenals
flupenthixol$_{GB}$	Depixol$_{GB}$, Fluanxol$_{GB}$, used for psychoses and related disorders
fluphenazine$_{GB,US}$	Modecate$_{GB}$, used for psychoses and related disorders
flurazepam$_{GB,US}$	Dalmane$_{GB,US}$, benzodiazepine hypnotic and anxiolytic
flurbiprofen$_{GB}$	Froben$_{GB}$, NSAID analgesic
Fortagesic$_{GB}$	compound analgesic containing pentazocine and paracetamol
Fortral$_{GB}$	*see pentazocine*$_{GB,US}$
fosfestrol$_{GB}$	Honvan$_{GB}$, converted to stilboestrol; used in malignant disease, e.g. prostatic carcinoma
framycetin$_{GB}$	Soframycin$_{GB}$, almost identical to neomycin in its actions and uses
Franol$_{GB}$	bronchodilator with sedation, contains ephedrine$_{GB,US}$, theophylline$_{GB,US}$ and phenobarbitone$_{GB,US}$
Frisium$_{GB}$	*see clobazam*$_{GB}$
Froben$_{GB}$	*see flurbiprofen*$_{GB}$
Frumil$_{GB}$	*amiloride*$_{GB,US}$ + *frusemide*$_{GB,US}$, combination diuretic
frusemide$_{GB,US}$	Lasix$_{GB,US}$, powerful loop diuretic, oral erosions have been reported
Fucidin$_{GB}$	*see sodium fusidate*$_{GB}$
Fulcin$_{GB}$	*see griseofulvin*$_{GB,US}$
Fulvicin$_{US}$	*see griseofulvin*$_{GB,US}$
Fungilin$_{GB}$	*see amphotericin*$_{GB,US}$
Fungizone$_{GB,US}$	*see amphotericin*$_{GB,US}$
Furadantin$_{GB,US}$	*see nitrofurantoin*$_{GB,US}$

furosemide$_{US}$	Lasix$_{GB,US}$, loop diuretic, oral erosions have been reported
Fybogel$_{GB}$	*see ispaghula husk*$_{GB}$
gamma benzene hexachloride$_{GB,US}$	treatment of lice and for scabies
Garamycin$_{GB,US}$	*see gentamicin*$_{GB,US}$
Gastrocote$_{GB}$	compound antacid
Gastrozepin$_{GB}$	*see pirenzepine*$_{GB}$
Gaviscon$_{GB,US}$	compound antacid containing alginic acid antacids and sucrose, can increase caries
Gelusil$_{GB,US}$	compound antacid
gentamicin$_{GB,US}$	Genticin$_{GB}$, Garamycin$_{GB,US}$, most important aminoglycoside antibiotic, broad spectrum; may cause renal and hepatic damage if blood levels become too high
Genticin$_{GB}$	*see gentamicin*$_{GB,US}$
glibenclamide$_{GB}$	oral hypoglycaemic agent, potentiated by aspirin
Glibenese$_{GB}$	*see glipizide*$_{GB,US}$
glipizide$_{GB,US}$	Glibenese$_{GB}$, Glucotrol$_{US}$, oral hypoglycaemic agent
Glucophage$_{GB}$	*see metformin*$_{GB}$
glyceryl trinitrate$_{GB,US}$	vasodilator, commonly used for angina pectoris
griseofulvin$_{GB,US}$	Fulcin$_{GB}$, Fulvicin$_{US}$, antifungal agent used for severe dermatophyte infections, may cause loss of taste and a disulfiram reaction with alcohol
Grisovin$_{GB}$	*see griseofulvin*$_{GB,US}$
guanethidine$_{GB,US}$	Ismelin$_{GB,US}$, adrenergic neurone-blocking agent used for hypertension, hypotensive effect of general anaesthetics potentiated, may cause parotid gland discomfort
Halcion$_{GB,US}$	*see triazolam*$_{GB,US}$
haloperidol$_{GB,US}$	Serenace$_{GB}$, used in acute and chronic schizophrenia and related disorders
Harmogen$_{GB}$	*see piperazine oestrone sulphate*$_{GB,US}$
Heminevrin$_{GB}$	*see chlormethiazole*$_{GB}$
heparin$_{GB,US}$	anticoagulant
heroin$_{GB}$	*see diamorphine*$_{GB}$

Herpid$_{GB}$	*see idoxuridine*$_{GB}$; Herpid is a colourless solution containing 5% idoxuridine in 100% dimethyl sulphoxide
hexochlorophane$_{GB,US}$	a germicide for external use, active against Gram-positive organisms
Hexopal$_{GB}$	*see inositol nicotinate*$_{GB,US}$
Hiprex$_{GB,US}$	*see hexamine*$_{GB,US}$
Hismanal$_{GB}$	*see astemizole*$_{GB}$
homatropine$_{GB,US}$	mydriatic
Honvan$_{GB}$	*see fosfestrol*$_{GB}$
Hydergine$_{GB,US}$	*see co-dergocrine mesylate*$_{GB,US}$
hydralazine$_{GB,US}$	Apresoline$_{GB,US}$, hypotensive agent active on the central nervous system; may give rise to a rheumatoid arthritis-like syndrome or sometimes a picture resembling disseminated lupus erythematosus
Hydrea$_{GB}$	*see hydroxyurea*$_{GB,US}$
hydrochlorothiazide$_{GB,US}$	Hydrosaluric$_{GB}$, also contained in Moduretic, Co-Betaloc, Dyazide, and Hydromet; a diuretic used for mild hypertension
hydrocortisone$_{GB,US}$	Cortisol$_{GB}$, the principal naturally occurring steroid. The soluble salt (hydrocortisone sodium succinate) can be given intravenously for rapid effect in an emergency. A suspension of the insoluble hydrocortisone acetate can be given intramuscularly for prolonged effect, and also intra-articularly
hydroflumethiazide$_{GB,US}$	Aldactide$_{GB}$, in combination with spironolactone, a thiazide diuretic
Hydromet$_{GB}$	*see methyldopa*$_{GB,US}$
Hydrosaluric$_{GB}$	*see hydrochlorothiazide*$_{GB,US}$
hydrotalcite$_{GB}$	Altacite$_{GB}$, antacid
hydroxocobalamin$_{GB}$	Neo-Cytamen$_{GB}$, vitamin B_{12}, given parenterally as maintenance therapy (usually 1 mg monthly)
hydroxychloroquine sulphate$_{GB,US}$	Plaquenil$_{GB,US}$, used in treatment of malaria, rheumatoid arthritis, and lupus erythematosus; can cause oral erosions
hydroxyurea$_{GB,US}$	Hydrea$_{GB}$, an orally active cytotoxic agent, probably acting by interfering with the synthesis of deoxyribonucleic

	acid, may cause bone marrow depression
Hygroton$_{GB,US}$	*see chlorthalidone*$_{GB,US}$
hyoscine$_{GB}$	*scopolamine*$_{US}$, chemically related to atropine; anticholinergic, used for its mydriatic and cycloplegic properties; may cause confusion
Hypnovase$_{GB}$	*see prazosin*$_{GB,US}$
Hypnovel$_{GB}$	*see midazolam*$_{GB,US}$
ibuprofen$_{GB,US}$	Brufen$_{GB}$, Nuprin$_{US}$, Motrin$_{GB,US}$, non-steroidal anti-inflammatory agent
idoxuridine$_{GB}$	Herpid$_{GB}$, antiviral agent
Isolone$_{GB,US}$	*see erythromycin*$_{GB,US}$
imipramine$_{GB,US}$	Tofranil$_{GB,US}$, tricyclic antidepressant, use local anaesthetics without adrenaline; may cause dryness of the mouth
Imodium$_{GB,US}$	*see loperamide*$_{GB,US}$
Imuran$_{GB,US}$	*see azathioprine*$_{GB,US}$
indapamide$_{GB,US}$	Natrilix$_{GB}$, Lozol$_{US}$, thiazide-like agent used for mild hypertension
Inderal$_{GB,US}$	*see propranolol*$_{GB,US}$
Indocid$_{GB}$	*see indomethacin*$_{GB,US}$
Indocin$_{US}$	*see indomethacin*$_{GB,US}$
indomethacin$_{GB,US}$	Indocid$_{GB}$, Indocin$_{US}$, non-steroidal anti-inflammatory agent; oral ulceration has been reported
Influvac$_{GB}$	influenza vaccine
Innovace$_{GB}$	*see enalapril maleate*$_{GB,US}$
inositol$_{GB,US}$	one of the vitamin B groups
insulin$_{GB,US}$	treatment of diabetes mellitus, salivary gland enlargement has been reported
insulin zinc suspension	intermediate-acting insulin
Intal$_{GB,US}$	*see sodium cromoglycate*$_{GB,US}$
Intropin$_{US}$	*see dopamine*$_{GB,US}$
ipecacuanha$_{GB,US}$	expectorant
ipratropium bromide$_{GB}$	Atrovent$_{GB}$, anticholinergic drug used for bronchospasm in chronic bronchitis
iproniazid$_{GB}$	Marsilid$_{GB}$, monoamine oxidase inhibitor used for depressive illness; amphetamine, ephedrine and opiate analgesics to be avoided

Ismelin$_{GB,US}$	*see guanethidine*$_{GB,US}$
isocarboxazid$_{GB,US}$	Marplan$_{GB,US}$, monoamine oxidase inhibitor used for depressive illness; amphetamine, ephedrine and opiate analgesics to be avoided
Isogel$_{GB}$	*see ispaghula husk*$_{GB}$
isoniazid$_{GB,US}$	Mynah$_{GB}$, antituberculous drug; interferes with the metabolism of vitamin B_6, may cause stomatitis, angular cheilitis, and oral ulceration
isophane	a combination of insulin and protamine
isoprenaline$_{GB}$	Saventrine$_{GB}$, sympathomimetic agent used in heart block and bronchospasm, can cause parotid swelling and oral ulceration, use local anaesthetics without adrenaline and avoid halothane
Isordil$_{GB,US}$	*see isosorbide dinitrate*$_{GB,US}$
isosorbide dinitrate$_{GB,US}$	Isordil$_{GB,US}$, long-acting nitrate used for angina
ispaghula husk$_{GB}$	Isogel$_{GB}$, Fybogel$_{GB}$, adsorbent agent used for diarrhoea
Jectofer$_{GB}$	injectable iron
Juvel$_{GB}$	multivitamin
kanamycin$_{GB,US}$	Kannasyn$_{GB}$, antibiotic for serious Gram-negative infections resistant to gentamicin; care needed with renal impairment
Kannasyn$_{GB}$	*see kanamycin*$_{GB,US}$
kaolin$_{GB,US}$	adsorbent antidiarrhoeal agent
Kaomycin$_{GB}$	*kaolin*$_{GB,US}$ + *neomycin*$_{GB,US}$
Kaopectate$_{GB,US}$	*see kaolin*$_{GB,US}$
Keflex$_{GB,US}$	*see cephalexin*$_{GB,US}$
Keflin$_{GB,US}$	*see cephalothin*$_{GB,US}$
Kefzol$_{GB,US}$	*see cephazolin*$_{GB}$
Kemadrin$_{GB}$	*see procyclidine*$_{GB,US}$
Kemicetine$_{GB}$	*see chloramphenicol*$_{GB,US}$
Kenalog in orobase$_{US}$	*see triamcinolone paste*$_{GB,US}$
ketoconazole$_{GB,US}$	Nizoral$_{GB,US}$, systemic fungicide; liable to cause liver damage
ketoprofen$_{GB,US}$	Alrheumat$_{GB}$, Orudis$_{GB,US}$, anti-inflammatory agent similar to ibuprofen

ketotifen$_{GB}$ Zaditen$_{GB}$, for prophylaxis in asthma, may cause a dry mouth

Kinidin$_{GB}$ *see quinidine*$_{GB,US}$

Kloref$_{GB}$ *see potassium chloride*$_{GB,US}$

Klorivess$_{US}$ *see potassium chloride*$_{GB,US}$

labetalol$_{GB}$ Trandate$_{GB}$, α- and β-adrenoceptor blocker for hypertension; potentiates hypotensive effect of general anaesthetics

lactulose$_{GB,US}$ Duphulac$_{GB}$, osmotic laxative used for constipation and in hepatic encephalopathy

Lanoxin$_{GB,US}$ *see digoxin*$_{GB,US}$

Largactil$_{GB}$ *see chlorpromazine*$_{GB,US}$

Lasikal$_{GB}$ *frusemide*$_{GB}$ + *potassium*$_{GB,US}$

Lasix$_{GB,US}$ *see frusemide*$_{GB}$ and *furosemide*$_{US}$

Ledercort$_{GB}$ *see triamcinolone*$_{GB,US}$

Lederfen$_{GB}$ *see fenbufen*$_{GB}$

Ledermycin$_{GB}$ *see demeclocycline*$_{GB,US}$

Lentizol$_{GB}$ *see amitriptyline*$_{GB,US}$

Leukeran$_{GB,US}$ *see chlorambucil*$_{GB,US}$

levodopa$_{GB,US}$ Madopar$_{GB}$, Sinemet$_{GB,US}$, dopaminergic drug used in parkinsonism; avoid use of halothane, serum levels increased with diazepam

Librax$_{US}$ *chlordiazepoxide*$_{GB,US}$ + *clidinium bromide*$_{GB,US}$

Libraxin$_{GB}$ *chlordiazepoxide*$_{GB,US}$ + *clidinium bromide*$_{GB,US}$

Librium$_{GB,US}$ *see chlordiazepoxide*$_{GB,US}$

Lidex$_{US}$ *see fluocinonide*$_{GB,US}$

Limbritol$_{GB,US}$ *see amitriptyline*$_{GB,US}$ + *chlordiazepoxide*$_{GB,US}$

Lincocin$_{GB,US}$ *see lincomycin*$_{GB,US}$

lincomycin$_{GB,US}$ Lincocin$_{GB,US}$, active against Gram-positive cocci, but use limited by serious side-effects, especially pseudomembranous colitis

lindane$_{GB}$ Lorexane$_{GB}$, for treatment of pediculosis and scabies

Lioresal$_{GB}$ *see baclofen*$_{GB,US}$

lithium carbonate$_{GB,US}$ Priadel$_{GB}$, prevention of mania and manic depressive illness, can cause hypothermia with diazepam

Lomotil$_{GB,US}$	*see diphenoxylate*$_{GB,US}$
lomustine$_{GB,US}$	CCNU$_{GB,US}$, cytotoxic agent, causes marrow depression
Loniten$_{GB}$	*see minoxidil*
loperamide$_{GB,US}$	Imodium$_{GB,US}$, antidiarrhoeal agent
Lopresor$_{GB,US}$	*see metoprolol*$_{GB,US}$
Lopurin$_{US}$	*see allopurinol*$_{GB,US}$
lorazepam$_{GB,US}$	Ativan$_{GB,US}$, benzodiazepine anxiolytic agent
Lorexane$_{GB}$	*see lindane*$_{GB}$
Loridine$_{US}$	*see cephaloridine*$_{GB,US}$
Luminal$_{GB,US}$	*see phenobarbitone*$_{GB,US}$
lysergic acid$_{GB}$	LSD – class A controlled drug
Maalox$_{GB,US}$	compound antacid
Madopar$_{GB}$	*levodopa*$_{GB,US}$ + *benserazide*$_{GB}$
Magnapen$_{GB}$	*ampicillin*$_{GB,US}$ + *flucloxacillin*$_{GB}$
magnesium trisilicate$_{GB,US}$	antacid
malathion$_{GB}$	Derbac$_{GB}$, used for lice and scabies infection
Maloprim$_{GB}$	*see pyrimethamine*$_{GB}$
Marcain$_{GB,US}$	*see bupivacaine*$_{GB,US}$
Marevan$_{GB}$	*see warfarin*$_{GB,US}$
Marplan$_{GB,US}$	*see isocarboxazid*$_{GB,US}$
Marsalid$_{GB}$	*see isoproniazid*$_{GB}$
Matulane$_{US}$	*see procarbazine*$_{GB,US}$
Maxolon$_{GB}$	*see metoclopramide*$_{GB,US}$
mebendazole$_{GB,US}$	Vermox$_{GB,US}$, for treatment of threadworm, roundworm and hookworm
mebeverine$_{GB}$	Colofac$_{GB}$, antispasmodic for colonic spasm
medazepam$_{GB}$	Nobrium$_{GB}$, anxiolytic
mefenamic acid$_{GB,US}$	Ponstan$_{GB}$, Ponstel$_{US}$, analgesic for mild to moderate pain, potentiates action of warfarin; avoid in patients with asthma or ulcerative colitis
mefruside$_{GB}$	Baycaron$_{GB}$, diuretic
Melleril$_{GB,US}$	*see thioridazine*$_{GB,US}$
melphalan$_{GB,US}$	Alkeran$_{GB,US}$, cytotoxic agent for myelomatosis, causes marrow depression
menadiol sodium phosphate$_{GB,US}$	Synkavit$_{GB,US}$, Synkayvite$_{US}$, vitamin K, water soluble by mouth or injection

mepacrine$_{GB}$	used for tapeworm infestation, known to cause oral erosions
meprobamate$_{GB,US}$	Equanil$_{GB,US}$, anxiolytic for mild anxiety
Merbentyl$_{GB}$	*see dicyclomine*$_{GB,US}$
mercaptopurine$_{GB,US}$	Puri-Nethol$_{GB}$, antimetabolite used in acute leukaemia, suppresses bone marrow
mesalazine$_{GB}$	Asacol$_{GB}$, used in ulcerative colitis where sulphasalazine intolerance exists
mersalyl$_{GB}$	mercurial diuretic
Mestinon$_{GB,US}$	*see pyridostigmine*$_{GB,US}$
mestranol$_{GB,US}$	present in sone oral contraceptives, occasionally cause light pigmentation in the mouth
metformin$_{GB}$	Glucophage$_{GB}$, biguanide oral hypoglycaemic agent
methadone$_{GB,US}$	Physeptone$_{GB}$, strong analgesic used in oral treatment of chronic pain in terminal disease, to be avoided in patients on monoamine oxidase inhibitors
methicillin$_{GB,US}$	parenteral penicillin for infections due to penicillinase-producing staphylococci
methimazole$_{US}$	Tapazole$_{US}$, treatment of hyperthyroidism, may cause loss of taste
methotrexate$_{GB,US}$	antimetabolite, depresses bone marrow, toxicity increased by aspirin
methyl cellulose$_{GB,US}$	bulk-forming laxative
methyldopa$_{GB,US}$	Aldomet$_{GB,US}$, hypotensive agent, can cause oral erosions and parotid discomfort
methylprednisolone$_{GB,US}$	glucocorticoid, suppresses adrenals
methysergide$_{GB,US}$	Deseril$_{GB}$, Sansent$_{US}$, antiserotinergic agent used in migraine and neuralgia
metoclopramide$_{GB,US}$	Maxolon$_{GB}$, Reglan$_{US}$, used for digestive disorders, speeds gastric emptying, used for nausea, but masseteric spasm and trismus have been reported as side-effects
metoprolol$_{GB,US}$	Betaloc$_{GB}$, Lopresor$_{GB,US}$, β-blocker, used for hypertension and angina, hypotensive effects of general anaesthetics potentiated
Metosyn$_{GB}$	*see fluocinonide*$_{GB,US}$
metronidazole$_{GB,US}$	Flagyl$_{GB,US}$, antimicrobial agent, highly active against anaerobic bacteria and

	protozoa. Potentiates action of warfarin. Should not be given during pregnancy or lactation or to patients being treated with disulfiram. Alcohol must be avoided
mexiletine$_{GB,US}$	Mexitil$_{GB}$, dysrhythmic agent used for ventricular arrhythmias
Mexitil$_{GB}$	*see mexiletine*$_{GB,US}$
mianserin$_{GB}$	Bolvidon$_{GB}$, tricyclic antidepressant, use local anaesthetics without adrenaline; leucopenia a rare side-effect
miconazole$_{GB,US}$	Daktarin$_{GB}$, Monistat$_{US}$, for fungal infections, topically or systemically
midazolam$_{GB,US}$	Hypnovel$_{GB}$, Versed$_{US}$, for sedation and amnesia
Midrin$_{GB,US}$	*see dichloralphenazone*$_{GB,US}$
Migraleve$_{GB}$	combination antimigraine preparation
Migravess$_{GB}$	combination antimigraine preparation
Migril$_{GB}$	*see ergotamine tartrate*$_{GB,US}$
Minipres$_{US}$	*see prazosin*$_{GB,US}$
minoxidil$_{GB,US}$	Loniten$_{GB,US}$, vasodilator hypotensive agent for severe hypertension; avoid general anaesthetics and use local anaesthetics without adrenaline
Mintec$_{GB}$	antispasmodic, antiflatulent agent for gastrointestinal disorders
mithramycin$_{GB,US}$	cytotoxic antibiotic useful for hypercalcaemia associated with malignancy; causes marked marrow depression
mitomycin$_{GB,US}$	cytotoxic antibiotic used for gastrointestinal tumours; causes marrow depression
Modecate$_{GB}$	*see fluphenazine*$_{GB,US}$
Moduretic$_{GB}$	*amiloride + hydrochlorothiazide*$_{GB,US}$
Mogadon$_{GB}$	*see nitrazepam*$_{GB}$
Monistat$_{US}$	*see miconazole*$_{GB,US}$
morphine$_{GB,US}$	opiate analgesic, not to be used in patients on monoamine oxidase inhibitors
Motilium$_{GB}$	*see domperidone*$_{GB}$
Motipress$_{GB}$	*fluphenazine*$_{GB,US}$ + *nortriptyline*$_{GB,US}$
Motival$_{GB}$	*fluphenazine*$_{GB,US}$ + *nortriptyline*$_{GB,US}$
MST 1$_{GB}$	oral preparation of morphine sulphate,

	not to be used on patients on monoamine oxidase inhibitors
Mucaine$_{GB}$	antacid
mustine$_{GB}$	alkylating drug particularly valuable in the treatment of Hodgkin's disease; depresses bone marrow
Mycardol$_{GB}$	*see pentaerythritol tetranitrate*$_{GB,US}$
Mycelex$_{US}$	*see clotrimazole*$_{GB,US}$
Mycostatin$_{US}$	*see nystatin*$_{GB,US}$
Mycota$_{GB}$	undecenoate fungicide
Myleran$_{GB,US}$	*see busulphan*$_{GB,US}$
Myocrisin$_{GB,US}$	*see sodium aurothiomalate*$_{GB,US}$
Mysoline$_{GB,US}$	*see primidone*$_{GB,US}$
Mysteclin$_{GB,US}$	*tetracycline + amphotericin B*$_{GB,US}$
Nacton$_{GB}$	*see poldine methylsulphate*$_{GB}$
nadolol$_{GB,US}$	Corgard$_{GB,US}$, β-blocker for angina and hypertension; hypotensive effect of general anaesthetics potentiated
nalbuphine hydrochloride$_{GB,US}$	Nubain$_{GB,US}$, opiate analgesic with minimal respiratory depression
Nalcrom$_{GB}$	*see sodium cromogylcate*$_{GB}$
nalidixic acid$_{GB,US}$	Negram$_{GB,US}$, urinary antibiotic
naloxone$_{GB,US}$	Narcan$_{GB,US}$, antidote to morphine-like drugs
nandrolone$_{GB,US}$	Durabolin$_{GB,US}$, anabolic steroid
Naprosyn$_{GB,US}$	*see naproxen*$_{GB,US}$
naproxen$_{GB,US}$	Naprosyn$_{GB,US}$, NSAID analgesic
Narcan$_{GB,US}$	*see naloxone*$_{GB,US}$
Nardil$_{GB,US}$	*see phenelzine*$_{GB,US}$
Natrilix$_{GB}$	*see indapamide*$_{GB}$
Natulan$_{GB}$	*see procarbazine*$_{GB,US}$
Navidrex$_{GB}$	*see cyclopenthiazide*$_{GB}$
nedocromil sodium$_{GB}$	Tilade$_{GB}$, asthma prophylactic
Nefopam$_{GB}$	Acupan$_{GB}$, powerful non-opiate analgesic
Negram$_{GB,US}$	*see nalidixic acid*$_{GB,US}$
Neo-Cytamen$_{GB}$	*see hydroxocobalamin*$_{GB}$
Neo-Mercazole$_{GB}$	*see carbimazole*$_{GB}$
neomycin$_{GB,US}$	non-parenteral aminoglycoside antibiotic
Neo-Naclex$_{GB}$	*see bendrofluazide*$_{GB}$
neostigmine$_{GB,US}$	anticholinesterase for diagnosis and treatment of myasthenia gravis

Nepenthe$_{GB}$	*see morphine*$_{GB,US}$
Netillin$_{GB}$	*see netilmicin*$_{GB,US}$
netilmicin$_{GB,US}$	Netillin$_{GB}$, Netromycin$_{US}$, antibiotic for Gram-negative infections resistant to gentamicin; general anaesthetics to be avoided
Netromycin$_{US}$	*see netilmicin*$_{GB,US}$
nicardipine$_{GB}$	Cardene$_{GB}$, calcium channel blocker, used in treatment of hypertension and angina
nifedipine$_{GB,US}$	Adalat$_{GB,US}$, used in treatment of angina, can cause gingival hyperplasia
nikethamide$_{GB,US}$	respiratory stimulant
nitrates$_{GB,US}$	for angina
nitrazepam$_{GB}$	Mogadon$_{GB}$, benzodiazepine sedative
nitrofurantoin$_{GB,US}$	Furadantin$_{GB,US}$, urinary antibiotic
Nitrolingual$_{GB}$	glyceryl trinitrate in a metered dose aerosol
Nivaquine$_{GB}$	*see chloroquine*$_{GB,US}$
nizatidine$_{GB}$	Axid$_{GB}$, H_2-receptor blocker for treatment of duodenal and gastric ulcer
Nizoral$_{GB,US}$	*see ketoconazole*$_{GB,US}$
noradrenaline$_{GB}$	Levophed$_{GB}$, a sympathomimetic amine
norethandrolone$_{GB}$	anabolic steroid
norethisterone$_{GB}$	sex hormone contraceptive, used in uterine dysfunction, occasionally causes light pigmentation in the mouth
Norgesic$_{GB,US}$	compound analgesic, avoid in patients with glaucoma
Normacol$_{GB}$	*see sterculia*$_{GB}$
nortriptyline$_{GB,US}$	tricyclic antidepressant, use local anaesthetics without adrenaline; may cause dryness of the mouth
Nubain$_{GB,US}$	*see nalbuphine hydrochloride*$_{GB}$
Nulacin$_{GB}$	antacid
Nutrizym$_{GB}$	pancreatic enzyme
nystatin$_{GB,US}$	Nystan$_{GB}$, Mycostatin$_{US}$, antifungal agent for candidiasis
Omnopon$_{GB}$	*see papaveretum*$_{GB}$
Oncovin$_{GB,US}$	*see vincristine*$_{GB,US}$
Optimax$_{GB}$	*see tryptophan*$_{GB}$
orciprenaline$_{GB}$	Alupent$_{GB}$, adrenoceptor stimulant for bronchospasm

orphenadrine$_{GB,US}$	Disipal$_{GB,US}$, for parkinsonism, anticholinergic
Orudis$_{GB,US}$	*see ketoprofen*$_{GB,US}$
ouabain$_{GB}$	cardiac glycoside for supraventricular dysrhythmias and heart failure
oxazepam$_{GB,US}$	short-acting anxiolytic
oxprenolol$_{GB}$	Trasicor$_{GB}$, β-blocker, hypotensive effect of general anaesthetics potentiated
oxymetazoline$_{GB,US}$	Afrazine$_{GB}$, Ilidine$_{GB}$, Alfrin$_{US}$, nasal drop decongestant; avoid in patients on monoamine oxidase inhibitors
oxymetholone$_{GB,US}$	Anapolon$_{GB}$, anabolic steroid
oxyphenbutazone$_{GB,US}$	Tanderil$_{GB}$, Tandearil$_{US}$, non-steroidal anti-inflammatory analgesic, may cause oral ulceration and enlargement of salivary glands
oxytetracycline$_{GB,US}$	tetracycline antibiotic
oxytocin$_{GB,US}$	Syntocinon$_{GB,US}$, myometrial stimulant
Palfium$_{GB}$	*see dextromoramide*$_{GB}$
Paludrine$_{GB}$	*see proguanil*$_{GB}$
Panadol$_{GB}$	*see paracetamol*$_{GB}$
Pancrease$_{US}$	pancreatic enzyme
Pancrex$_{GB}$	pancreatic enzyme
papaveretum$_{GB}$	Omnopon$_{GB}$, opiate analgesic, avoid in patients on monoamine oxidase inhibitors
paracetamol$_{GB}$	Panadol$_{GB}$, mild analgesic, overdosage may lead to severe liver damage, potentiated by metoclopramide
paraldehyde$_{GB,US}$	occasionally used for status epilepticus
Paramax$_{GB}$	combined preparation for migraine containing paracetamol and metoclopramide
Parlodel$_{GB,US}$	*see bromocriptine*$_{GB,US}$
Parnate$_{GB,US}$	*see tranylcypromine*$_{GB,US}$
Pavulon$_{GB,US}$	*see pancuronium*$_{GB,US}$
Penbritin$_{GB}$	*see ampicillin*$_{GB,US}$
penicillamine$_{GB,US}$	used in active rheumatoid arthritis, Wilson's disease and cystinuria; may cause loss of taste and oral manifestation of pemphigus
penicillin$_{GB,US}$	bactericidal antibiotic

pentaerythritol$_{GB,US}$	Mycardol$_{GB}$, prophylaxis of angina
pentazocine$_{GB,US}$	Fortral$_{GB}$, Talwin$_{US}$, analgesic for moderate to severe pain
pentobarbitone	a barbiturate hypnotic, now seldom used
Pepsid$_{GB}$	*see famotidine*$_{GB}$
perhexiline maleate$_{GB}$	for angina
Periactin$_{GB,US}$	*see cyproheptadine*$_{GB,US}$
Peritrate$_{GB,US}$	*see pentaerythritol tetranitrate*$_{GB,US}$
perphenazine$_{GB,US}$	Fentazin$_{GB}$, antinausea, also schizophrenia and related psychoses
Persantin$_{GB,US}$	*see dipyridamole*$_{GB,US}$
pethidine$_{GB}$	opiate analgesic, avoid in patients on monoamine oxidase inhibitors
phenacetin$_{GB,US}$	analgesic; prolonged use leads to serious renal damage
phenelzine$_{GB,US}$	Nardil$_{GB,US}$, monoamine oxidase inhibitor for depressive illness; amphetamine, ephedrine and opiate analgesics to be avoided
Phenergan$_{GB,US}$	*see promethazine*$_{GB,US}$
phenindione$_{GB}$	Dindevan$_{GB}$, anticoagulant; assess clotting time before extractions
pheniramine maleate$_{GB,US}$	Daneral$_{GB}$, antihistamine
phenobarbitone$_{GB,US}$	barbiturate little used now as a sedative, but occasionally used in epilepsy
phenoperidine$_{GB}$	used for analgesia in operations
phenoxybenzamine$_{GB,US}$	Dibenyline$_{GB}$, Dibenzyline$_{US}$, α-adrenergic blocker used to control hypertension in phaeochromocytomata
Phensedyl$_{GB}$	cough linctus
phentolamine$_{GB,US}$	Regitine$_{US}$, Rogitine$_{GB}$, α-adrenergic blocker; indications as for phenoxybenzamine
phenylbutazone$_{GB,US}$	Butazolidin$_{GB,US}$, non-steroidal anti-inflammatory analgesic; may cause serious gastrointestinal haemorrhage, and oral ulceration and parotid enlargement
phenylephrine$_{GB,US}$	sympathomimetic agent for hypotension and used in eye drops as a mydriatic
phenytoin$_{GB,US}$	Epanutin$_{GB}$, Dilantin$_{US}$, anti-epileptic, frequently causes gingival hyperplasia and occasionally lupus erythematosus syndrome or erythema multiforme,

	action potentiated by diazepam and aspirin
Phyllocontin$_{GB,US}$	*see aminophylline*$_{GB,US}$
Physeptone$_{GB}$	*see methadone*$_{GB,US}$
physostigmine$_{GB,US}$	anticholinesterase used as a miotic
pilocarpine$_{GB,US}$	miotic
pindolol$_{GB,US}$	Visken$_{GB,US}$, β-adrenergic blocker, hypotensive effect of general anaesthetic potentiated
piperacillin$_{GB,US}$	Pipril$_{GB}$, Pipracil$_{US}$, antibiotic for severe infections caused by Gram-positive and Gram-negative anaerobic bacteria
piperazine$_{GB}$	Pripsen$_{GB}$, antihelminthic for threadworm and roundworm infestations
piperazine oestrone sulphate$_{GB,US}$	Harmogen$_{GB}$, an oestrogen
pirenzepine$_{GB}$	Gastrozepin$_{GB}$, selective anticholinergic drug used to heal peptic ulcers
Piriton$_{GB}$	*see chlorpheniramine*$_{GB,US}$
piroxicam$_{GB}$	Feldene$_{GB}$, NSAID analgesic
pivampicillin	*Miraxid*$_{GB}$, *broad-spectrum antibiotic*
pizotifen$_{GB}$	Sanomigran$_{GB}$, for migraine prophylaxis
Plaquenil$_{GB,US}$	*see hydroxychloroquine*$_{GB,US}$
podophyllum$_{GB}$	Podophyllin Paint$_{GB}$, used for treatment of warts
poldine$_{GB}$	Nacton$_{GB}$, antispasmodic used in peptic ulcer and spastic colon
polymyxin$_{GB,US}$	antibiotic effective against Gram-negative organisms
Ponderax$_{GB}$	*see fenfluramine*$_{GB,US}$
Pondimin$_{US}$	*see fenfluramine*$_{GB,US}$
Ponstan$_{GB}$	*see mefenamic acid*$_{GB,US}$
potassium citrate$_{GB,US}$	for alkalinizing urine
practolol$_{GB}$	β-adrenergic blocker; serious side effects limit its use to short-term treatment of dysrhythmias; hypotensive effects of general anaesthetics potentiated, oral erosions reported
prazosin$_{GB,US}$	Hypovase$_{GB}$, Minipress$_{US}$, potent vasodilator hypotensive agent, may potentiate hypotensive effect of general anaesthetics
prednisolone$_{GB,US}$	corticosteroid, may suppress adrenals
Pregaday$_{GB}$	iron + folate

Prestim$_{GB}$	*timolol*$_{GB,US}$ + *bendrofluazide*$_{GB}$
Priadel$_{GB}$	*see lithium carbonate*$_{GB,US}$
primaquine$_{GB,US}$	used to eradicate benign tertian malaria
primidone$_{GB,US}$	Mysoline$_{GB,US}$, for tonic, clonic, and partial seizures
Primperan$_{GB}$	*see metoclopramide*$_{GB,US}$
Pripsen$_{GB}$	*see piperazine*$_{GB}$
Pro-Banthine$_{GB,US}$	*see propantheline bromide*$_{GB,US}$
probenecid$_{GB,US}$	Benemid$_{GB,US}$, uricosuric agent; reduces renal excretion of penicillin; aspirin to be avoided
procainamide$_{GB,US}$	Pronestyl$_{GB}$, anti-arrhythmia agent; may cause lupus erythematosus syndrome
procarbazine$_{GB,US}$	Natulan$_{GB}$, Matulane$_{US}$, cytotoxic agent used in combination therapy for Hodgkin's disease, causes marrow depression
prochlorperazine$_{GB,US}$	Stemetil$_{GB}$, Compazine$_{US}$, for nausea and vertigo
procyclidine$_{GB,US}$	Kemadrin$_{GB,US}$, anticholinergic drug used for parkinsonism
proguanil$_{GB}$	Paludrine$_{GB}$, for prophylaxis against malaria; known to cause oral ulceration
Proloprim$_{US}$	*see trimethoprim*$_{GB,US}$
promazine$_{GB}$	Sparine$_{GB,US}$, for mild psychiatric disturbances in the elderly
promethazine$_{GB,US}$	Phenergan$_{GB,US}$, antihistamine
Propaderm$_{GB}$	*see beclomethasone dipropionate*$_{GB,US}$
propantheline bromide$_{GB,US}$	Pro-Banthine$_{GB,US}$, anticholinergic agent; may cause a dry mouth
propoxyphene napsylate$_{US}$	Darvocet-N$_{US}$, medium strength analgesic
propranolol$_{GB,US}$	Inderal$_{GB,US}$, β-adrenergic blocker, hypotensive effect of general anaesthetics potentiated; use local anaesthetics without adrenaline
propylthiouracil$_{GB,US}$	used in the treatment of hyperthyroidism
Prostigmin$_{GB,US}$	*see neostigmine*$_{GB,US}$
Prothiaden$_{GB}$	*see dothiepin*$_{GB}$
protriptyline$_{GB,US}$	tricyclic antidepressant with stimulant action, use local anaesthetics without adrenaline
Pyopen$_{GB,US}$	*see carbenicillin*$_{GB,US}$

pyrazinamide$_{GB}$	Zinamide$_{GB}$, antituberculous antibiotic
pyridostigmine$_{GB,US}$	Mestinon$_{GB,US}$, anticholinesterase used for myasthenia gravis
pyrimethamine$_{GB,US}$	Daraprim$_{GB,US}$, Fansidar$_{GB}$, chemoprophylaxis of malaria
Pyrogastrone$_{GB}$	compound antacid
Questran$_{GB,US}$	*see cholestyramine*$_{GB,US}$
quinidine$_{GB,US}$	used for supraventricular tachycardias; can cause oral erosions
quinine$_{GB,US}$	used for malignant tertian malaria and muscular cramps
ranitidine$_{GB,US}$	Zantac$_{GB,US}$, H_2-receptor antagonist for treatment of dyspeptic conditions
Rapitard$_{GB}$	*see insulin*$_{GB,US}$
Rastinon$_{GB}$	*see tolbutamide*$_{GB,US}$
rauwolfia$_{GB,US}$	hypotensive agent
reserpine$_{GB,US}$	Serpasil$_{GB,US}$, hypotensive agent
Retrovir$_{GB}$	*see zidovudine*$_{GB}$
Rheumox$_{GB}$	*see azapropazone*$_{GB}$
rifampicin$_{GB}$	first-line treatment of tuberculosis
rifampin$_{US}$	first-line treatment of tuberculosis
Rivotril$_{GB}$	*see clonazepam*$_{GB,US}$
Rynacrom$_{GB}$	*see sodium cromogylcate*$_{GB}$, nasal insufflation
Rythmodan$_{GB}$	*see disopyramide*$_{GB,US}$
Salazopyrin$_{GB,US}$	*see sulphasalazine*$_{GB,US}$
salbutamol$_{GB}$	Ventolin$_{GB}$, β-adrenoceptor stimulant for bronchospasm
Salivix$_{GB}$	an artificial saliva which contains buffered malic acid, is sugar free and stimulates salivation
Sandimmun$_{US}$	*see cyclosporin*$_{GB,US}$
Sandocal$_{GB}$	calcium preparation
Sanomigran$_{GB}$	*see pizotifen*$_{GB,US}$
Sansert$_{US}$	*see methysergide*$_{GB,US}$
Sanset$_{US}$	*see methysergide*$_{GB,US}$
Saventrine$_{GB}$	*see isoprenaline*$_{GB}$
Sectral$_{GB,US}$	*see acebutolol*$_{GB,US}$
Septra$_{US}$	*see co-trimoxazole*$_{GB,US}$
Septrin$_{GB}$	*see co-trimoxazole*$_{GB,US}$
Serc$_{GB}$	*see betahistine*$_{GB}$

Serenace$_{GB}$	*see haloperidol*$_{GB,US}$
Serpasil$_{GB,US}$	*see reserpine*$_{GB,US}$
Sinemet$_{GB,US}$	*see levodopa*$_{GB,US}$
Sodium amytal$_{GB}$	*see amylobarbitone sodium*$_{GB}$
sodium aurothiomalate$_{GB}$	Myocrisin$_{GB}$, for treatment of severe rheumatoid arthritis
sodium cromoglycate$_{GB}$	Intal$_{GB}$, cell membrane stabilizer used as prophylactic agent in asthma
sodium fusidate$_{GB}$	Fucidine$_{GB}$, narrow-spectrum antibiotic used for penicillin-resistant staphylococci
sodium nitroprusside$_{GB,US}$	Nipride$_{GB,US}$, used as intravenous infusion in hypertensive crises
sodium valproate$_{GB}$	Epilim$_{GB}$ used for tonic–clonic fits
Soframycin$_{GB}$	*see framycetin sulphate*$_{GB}$
Soneryl$_{GB}$	*see butobarbitone*$_{GB,US}$
Sotacor$_{GB}$	*see sotalol*$_{GB}$
sotalol$_{GB}$	Sotacor$_{GB}$, β-adrenoceptor blocker, hypotensive effect of general anaesthetics potentiated
Spasmonal$_{GB}$	intestinal antispasmodic
Sparine$_{GB,US}$	*see promazine*$_{GB}$
spironolactone$_{GB,US}$	Aldactone$_{GB,US}$, aldosterone antagonist; weak diuretic useful in oedematous states
stanozolol$_{GB,US}$	Stromba$_{GB}$, anabolic steroid
Stelazine$_{GB,US}$	*see trifluoperazine*$_{GB,US}$
Stemetil$_{GB}$	*see prochlorperazine*$_{GB,US}$
sterculia$_{GB}$	Normacol$_{GB}$, bulk laxative
stilboestrol$_{GB}$	female sex hormone used in treatment of prostatic carcinoma
streptomycin$_{GB}$	first-line drug for tuberculosis; serious side-effects, ototoxicity and nephrotoxicity
Stromba$_{GB}$	*see stanozolol*$_{GB,US}$
Stugeron$_{GB}$	*see cinnarizine*$_{GB}$
sucralfate$_{GB,US}$	Antepsin$_{GB}$, Carafate$_{US}$, ulcer healing agent
sulindac$_{GB,US}$	Clinoral$_{GB,US}$, NSAID analgesic
sulphacetamide$_{GB,US}$	sulphonamide for eye infections
sulphadiazine$_{GB,US}$	sulphonamide used for meningococcal meningitis

sulphadimidine$_{GB}$	sulphonamide for urinary tract infections
sulphamethizole$_{GB,US}$	sulphonamide for urinary tract infections
sulphasalazine$_{GB,US}$	Salazopyrin$_{GB,US}$, for treatment of ulcerative colitis
sulphinopyrazone$_{GB,US}$	Anturan$_{GB,US}$, antiplatelet drug used for prophylaxis after myocardial infarctions
Surmontil$_{GB,US}$	*see trimipramine*$_{GB,US}$
Sustac$_{GB}$	*see glyceryl trinitrate*$_{GB,US}$
Symmetrel$_{GB,US}$	*see amantadine*$_{GB,US}$
Synacthen$_{GB}$	*see tetracosactrin*$_{GB}$
Tagamet$_{GB,US}$	*see cimetidine*$_{GB,US}$
talampicillin$_{GB}$	Talpen$_{GB}$, ester of ampicillin rapidly absorbed from the gut, may effect adsorption of oral contraceptives
Talpen$_{GB}$	*see talampicillin*$_{GB,US}$
Talwin$_{US}$	*see pentazocine*$_{GB,US}$
tamoxifen$_{GB,US}$	Nolvadex$_{GB,US}$, anti-oestrogen for breast cancer
Tanderil$_{GB,US}$	*see oxyphenbutazone*$_{GB,US}$
Tegopen$_{US}$	*see cloxacillin*$_{GB,US}$
Tegretol$_{GB,US}$	*see carbamazepine*$_{GB,US}$
temazepam$_{GB,US}$	Normison$_{GB}$, Restoril$_{US}$, benzodiazepine hypnotic and sedative
Temgesic$_{GB}$	*see buprenorphine*$_{GB,US}$
Tenoretic$_{GB,US}$	*atenolol*$_{GB,US}$ + *chlorthalidone*$_{GB,US}$
Tenormin$_{GB,US}$	*see atenolol*$_{GB,US}$
Tenuate$_{GB,US}$	*see diethylpropion*$_{GB,US}$
terbutaline$_{GB,US}$	Bricanyl$_{GB,US}$, β-adrenoceptor stimulant for bronchospasm
terfenadine$_{GB,US}$	Triludan$_{GB}$, Seldane$_{US}$, antihistamine
Terramycin$_{GB,US}$	*see oxytetracycline*$_{GB,US}$
tetracosactrin$_{GB}$	Synacthen$_{GB}$, adrenal stimulant
tetracycline$_{GB,US}$	broad-spectrum antibiotic useful in treatment of *Rickettsia* and *Mycoplasma*; to be avoided in pregnancy and in children
theophylline$_{GB,US}$	Neulin$_{GB}$, xanthine derivative used for bronchospasm
thioguanine$_{GB,US}$	Lanvis$_{GB}$, antimetabolite for acute leukaemias, causes marrow depression
thioridazine$_{GB,US}$	Melleril$_{GB}$, antipsychotic drug
thiotepa$_{GB,US}$	alkylating agent for malignant effusions

thyroxine$_{GB,US}$	Eltroxin$_{GB}$, Synthroid$_{US}$, thyroid hormone for replacement therapy in hypothyroidism
Tilade$_{GB}$	*see nedocromil sodium*$_{GB}$
timolol$_{GB,US}$	Blocadren$_{GB}$, β-adrenoceptor blocker for hypertension and angina; hypotensive effect of general anaesthetics potentiated
tobramycin$_{GB,US}$	Nebcin$_{GB}$, aminoglycoside for treatment of pseudomonas infections
tocainide$_{GB,US}$	Tonocard$_{GB,US}$, used in acute ventricular arrhythmias; neutropenia and agranulocytosis reported
Tofranil$_{GB,US}$	*see imipramine*$_{GB,US}$
tolbutamide$_{GB,US}$	Rastinon$_{GB}$, sulphonylurea used as hypoglycaemic in diabetes, potentiated by oral aspirin; has been known to cause oral erosions
Trandate$_{GB,US}$	*see labetalol*$_{GB,US}$
tranexamic acid$_{GB}$	Cyklokapron$_{GB}$, antifibrinolytic agent used for haemorrhage after prostatectomy and/or haemophiliacs
Tranxene$_{GB,US}$	*see clorazepate*$_{GB}$
tranylcypromine$_{GB,US}$	Parnate$_{GB,US}$, monoamine oxidase inhibitor for depressive illness; amphetamine, ephedrine and opiate analgesics to be avoided
Trasicor$_{GB}$	*see oxprenolol*$_{GB}$
Trasidrex$_{GB}$	*oxprenolol*$_{GB}$ + *cyclopenthiazide*$_{GB}$
Trasylol$_{GB}$	*see aprotinin*$_{GB}$
triamcinolone$_{GB,US}$	Adcortyl$_{GB}$, Kenalog$_{GB,US}$, corticosteroid
triamterene$_{GB,US}$	Dyazide$_{GB,US}$, Dytac$_{GB}$, for oedema and potassium conservation with thiazide and loop diuretics
triazolam$_{GB}$	Halcion$_{GB}$, hypnotic and sedative
trifluoperazine$_{GB,US}$	Stelazine$_{GB,US}$, for schizophrenia and related psychoses
trimeprazine$_{GB,US}$	Vallergan$_{GB}$, antipruritic agent
trimethoprim$_{GB,US}$	Monotrim$_{GB}$, Proloprim$_{US}$, broad-spectrum antibiotic
trimipramine$_{GB,US}$	Surmontil$_{GB,US}$, tricyclic antidepressant with sedative properties, use local anaesthetics without adrenaline
tripotassium dicitratobismuthate$_{GB}$	De-Nol$_{GB}$, ulcer healing agent

Tryptizol$_{GB}$	*see amitriptyline*$_{GB,US}$
tryptophan$_{GB,US}$	Optimax$_{GB}$, antidepressant
Tylenol$_{US}$	*see acetaminophen*$_{US}$
Ultratard$_{GB}$	slow-onset, long-acting insulin
Urispas$_{GB,US}$	*see flavoxate*$_{GB,US}$
ursodeoxycholic acid$_{GB}$	for dissolution of cholesterol gallstones
Valium$_{GB,US}$	*see diazepam*$_{GB,US}$
Vallergan$_{GB}$	*see trimeprazine*$_{GB,US}$
valproic acid$_{US}$	Depokene$_{US}$, used for petit mal
vancomycin$_{GB,US}$	Vancocin$_{GB}$, bactericidal antibiotic used for the treatment of pseudomembranous colitis
Vanceril$_{US}$	beclomethasone inhaler
Vascardin$_{GB}$	*see isosorbide*$_{GB,US}$
vasopressin$_{GB,US}$	antidiuretic hormone; treatment for diabetes insipidus
Velban$_{US}$	*see vinblastine*$_{GB,US}$
Velbe$_{GB}$	*see vinblastine*$_{GB,US}$
Velosef$_{GB,US}$	*see cephradine*$_{GB,US}$
Ventolin$_{GB,US}$	*see salbutamol*$_{GB,US}$
verapamil$_{GB,US}$	Cordilox$_{GB}$, Calan$_{US}$, used for supraventricular arrhythmias
Vermox$_{GB}$	*see mebendazole*$_{GB}$
Versed$_{US}$	*see midazolam*$_{GB,US}$
Vibramycin$_{GB}$	*see doxycycline*$_{GB}$
vinblastine$_{GB,US}$	Velbe$_{GB}$, Velban$_{US}$, vinca alkaloid for management of lymphomata; causes bone marrow depression
vincristine$_{GB,US}$	Oncovin$_{GB,US}$, vinca alkaloid, major drug in management of lymphomata and leukaemia; causes marrow depression
Viskaldix$_{GB}$	*pindolol*$_{GB}$ + *clopamide*$_{GB}$
Voltarol$_{GB}$	*see diclofenac*$_{GB}$
warfarin$_{GB,US}$	Marevan$_{GB}$, Coumadin$_{US}$, anticoagulant, potentiated by many drugs, including aspirin, mefenamic acid, metronidazole, cimetidine and also alcohol
Welldorm$_{GB}$	*see dichloralphenazone*$_{GB,US}$

xylometazoline$_{GB,US}$	Otrivine$_{GB}$, Otrivin$_{US}$, nasal decongestant, to be avoided in patients on monoamine oxidase inhibitors
Zaditen$_{GB}$	*see ketotifen*$_{GB}$
Zantac$_{GB,US}$	*see ranitidine*$_{GB,US}$
Zarontin$_{GB,US}$	*see ethosuximide*$_{GB,US}$
Zinacef$_{GB}$	*see cefuroxime*$_{GB}$
Zinamide$_{GB}$	*see pyrazinamide*$_{GB}$
Zyloprim$_{US}$	*see allopurinol*$_{GB,US}$
Zyloric$_{GB}$	*see allopurinol*$_{GB,US}$
zidovudine$_{GB}$	Retrovir$_{GB}$, for treatment of AIDS and ARC
Zovirax$_{GB,US}$	*see acyclovir*$_{GB,US}$